WHAT PEOPLE ARE SAYING ABOUT LISA STRINGER AND *GOD DID NOT DO THIS TO ME...*

Perspective changes not with words, but with life's challenges encountered. What we take for granted can be stripped away with one doctor's diagnosis. In her book, Lisa Stringer shares her own journey of realization, not as the patient, but as the wife of the one who experienced the diagnosis of Stage 4 cancer. I believe this will not only encourage family members but be a great tool for all who are navigating the roadblocks of life.

—*Joni Lamb*
Co-founder, Daystar Television Network

I just finished reading *God Did Not Do This to Me* and felt it was well written. I enjoyed reading it and could see (and feel) the hand of God through your family battle and journey with cancer then remission. A good writer makes you feel as if you were there during the story line, and Lisa Stringer came through in that area. Your testimony will continue to be a great source of encouragement to many as you share your story of faith, commitment, and God's grace with those in need.

—*Alan Bullock*
Vice president, Daystar Television Network

The chronicle of this journey moved me deeply because I have witnessed this priceless family minister through this personal trial with a tangible, authentic consistent witness in every place to every face, every time. The love and reality of God was shared with everyone in their path: medica'
friends, associates, and strangers.
for all to know the Lord personally
this testimony. Furthermore, the

their nation and world even though in this health battle. Their eyes were stayed on the Lord to overcome. "So help me God" is a theme throughout this story as this family leaned upon the truth of Scripture—the living Word of God Himself—and kept their radar focused on the Lord Jesus Christ. This is a call to believers everywhere to fast and intercede for our fellow brothers and sisters in need. Whether a health crisis or another battle, this journey will lead you to seek the Lord for your own victory! I thank God for His kingdom increase through the healing of Doug and grace to his family—so that privilege of the irrevocable call of God flies on like the eagle.

—*Lisa Crump*
Vice president, Volunteer Mobilization
and Liaison to Prayer Ministries
National Day of Prayer Task Force

The unexpected crisis in life comes to all of us without warning or time to prepare. That is why this book is a must read! It will encourage, give hope, and help to those who are currently trying to maneuver the hairpin curve of crisis and it will help those whose road is currently smooth and straight to now make large deposits of faith and trust in our God who will see all of us through the good, bad, and impossible moments of this life. Thank you for sharing what it means to walk by faith and not by sight!

—*Becky Riggle*
Grace Community Church, Houston, Texas

Little did I know that day in July 2002 that God gifted me with an apostolic father of the faith, Pastor Doug Stringer. My personal life and ministry has been impacted on so many levels. Lisa Stringer is a woman of strength, humility, and courage, a woman whose life reflects her abandoned love and servant's heart for her heavenly Father and her family. I am honored to call her friend! Thank you, Lisa, for writing this book, as the daughter of a father you lost to cancer, the daughter of a mother who lives life with you as a widow, and as a wife who walked the journey of battling cancer with her husband. Many daughters have done well, but you excel as a beautiful example, of a hero of the faith, for all women to learn from your life! This book exemplifies biblical proportion faith. You faced the Red Sea and crossed over on dry ground. You put Christ and others first as you and your family fought the good fight together on every level of life:

+ In the spirit, with weapons of faith, prayer, communion, and obedience to your call to serve.

+ In the medical realm, with chemo and medicine.

+ In the soul, staying on top of and sorting through intense painful emotions.

+ In the natural, with exercise and dietary changes.

+ In the relational realm, by caring for one another through it all.

You gathered five smooth stones and, in the name of the Lord, the giant was slain! What a living testimony your family is of the love and power of God revealed through a life of obedience.

This book will touch the lives of multitudes who have had to confront the pain of loss on any level of life and especially those who are on the journey of battling a diagnosis of infirmity. I remember those days when the whole world was praying and believing for a miracle. As I would look at the magnet picture of Doug with his bald head on my refrigerator, one of my many prayers was, "Lord, Ashley prayed for a daddy. You didn't bless this child with Doug as her dada to now take him home to be with You. The prayers of this child have Your heart. I add my faith to hers and agree with Ashley! Daddy will live and testify of the goodness of the Lord in the land of the living! Whose report will you believe? I believe the report of the Lord!"

—*Marlene J. Yeo*
Director, Somebody Cares New England
Director, He Cares for Me
Pastor, CCF Ministries, Lowell, MA

How could a book about cancer be inspirational and faith-building? It's because Lisa Stringer's book focuses not on the power of cancer, but on the goodness of God and His faithful presence while we seem to be walking through *"the valley of the shadow of death"* (Psalm 23:4). Many people who receive a cancer diagnosis are overwhelmed by fear. Some immediately put their trust in medical science, as if God was no longer the Great Physician. Others reject medical options altogether, hoping for a divine miracle, but refusing to avail themselves of the help of doctors. Lisa Stringer's book is an honest account of the how the Stringer family sought the Lord's guidance each step of the way, ultimately experiencing profound victory amid gut-wrenching challenges. Whether you or a loved one is facing cancer or some other life-altering trial, you will be transformed by the hope and courage you find in these pages.

—*Jim Buchan*
Author, writer and speaker, Crosslink Ministries

The world so much starves for the lack of the real, day-to-day stories of those who have encountered troubles, even life-threatening assaults, and have experienced the transformative power and relief of the gospel. Lisa Stringer shares just such a personal and family story in her new book, *God Did Not Do This to Me.*

Her words of her personal and her family's struggles as her husband was diagnosed with stage-four cancer are reminiscent of the apostle Paul's incredible and palpable words in his letter to the Philippians. Therein, he describes his many struggles and agonies as a "*fellowship of* [Christ's] *sufferings,*" which led to such a valuable result in his life that far surpassed any and everything else that he as a human being could ever experience—that being "*knowing Christ Jesus* [his] *Lord!*" Lisa Stringer's story is just such a similar, transparent testimony. I heartily recommend everyone read and listen to her victorious battle!

—*Randall J. Pannell, PhD, MDiv*
Professor of Christian Ministry, North Greenville University

GOD DIDNOT DOTHIS TO ME

GOD DIDNOT DOTHIS TOME

*Finding Hope, Courage, and Faith
to Face Our Toughest Challenge*

LISA STRINGER

WHITAKER
HOUSE

GOD DID NOT DO THIS TO ME
Finding Hope, Courage, and Faith to Face Our Toughest Challenge

Somebody Cares International
P.O. Box 925489
Houston, TX 77292
www.tpmi.org
www.dougstringer.com
www.somebodycares.org

ISBN: 978-1-64123-455-9
eBook ISBN: 978-1-64123-456-6
Printed in the United States of America
© 2020 by Lisa Stringer

Whitaker House
1030 Hunt Valley Circle
New Kensington, PA 15068
www.whitakerhouse.com

Library of Congress Cataloging-in-Publication Data
LC record available at https://lccn.loc.gov/2020004295
LC ebook record available at https://lccn.loc.gov/2020004296

1 2 3 4 5 6 7 8 9 10 11 ⨆⨆ 27 26 25 24 23 22 21 20

DEDICATION

This book is dedicated to the many who have gone before us, who chose to give it their all when met by unexpected detours… some of whom are now rejoicing in the presence of the Lord. To everyone who joined our journey and contended for us in prayer, you were a vital part of our story and I thank God for you daily.

To my family, both spiritual and natural, and dearest friends, you know who you are and how much you mean to me. Thank you for never giving up and always speaking life over us.

Doug, thank you for fighting for us, for your destiny, and for reminding us that God did not do this to you; therefore, it didn't belong to you. You are the best thing that could have ever happened to me outside of my salvation. I love you more than words can express.

Ashley, you are joy, love, and faith to the max. Never lose that gift and keep changing the world one smile at a time.

When words fail me, my eyes fill with tears of gratitude to God for His provision, abounding love, mercy, and grace. I don't know how people live without Him. He makes all things work together for good.

CONTENTS

FOREWORD

During my sixteen years of treating patients with ear, nose, and throat disorders, I have diagnosed and treated many patients with head and neck cancers. The patients look to us for answers about their cancer. They ask, "Why me? How long has it been there? What are my survival odds? Why does God allow this?"

As a Christian, I have a foundational string of verses that I keep in the back of my mind when I have a conversation with someone who is asking, "Who is Jesus?" or "What is grace?" These Scriptures move through Romans—5:12 to 3:23 to 6:23 to 5:8—to Ephesians 2:8–10.

I keep these verses at the core of our conversation and cater the flavor of my words to the appropriate personality and place. As I have matured in my Christianity, this flow of verses keeps me from "shooting from the hip" when I have the opportunity to evangelize.

After reading Lisa's book, I was humbled by a profound realization. I "shoot from the hip" when providing spiritual insight to a cancer patient's questions. Even though I run a men's ministry and rely on Scripture to help disciple those needing spiritual growth, I did not have an intentional scriptural basis to provide responses to my patients' questions when they have head or neck cancers. Of course, the Holy Spirit was spilling over into my discussions with my cancer patients, but would you consider that maybe at a subconscious level I resisted it? Hear this: I received my surgical training before accepting Christ as my Savior at the age of thirty-six. I was trained to give objective diagnostic and therapeutic information to patients prior to realizing the depth and power of God's grace and omnipotence. I had not received *any* training on the application of Scripture to this process. I had not read a book that correlated grace into the unique issues of patients battling death. But God has provided that book now.

After reading *God Did Not Do This to Me*, I have purposeful Scripture to rely on and use as the core of my conversation when addressing these precious patients' fears and despair during the seemingly endless sequence of events that accompany cancer diagnosis and treatments. Lisa Stringer's book has been my sanctifying grace continuing medical education.

This book is packed with relevant Scripture that perfectly applies to every step of the roller coaster ride of emotions and spiritual attacks that a cancer patient has to endure. It is a *must read* for every physician and health care provider who interacts with cancer patients. Christ was very intentional about His pursuit of our salvation. As health care providers acting as the hands and feet of Christ through Christian action, we are called to be intentional in our responses to these patients. We do not receive this type of training during residency and I don't recall any courses at our annual medical education meetings that provide the information that I obtained from this book.

Thank you, God, for using Lisa to deliver your sanctifying grace to me!

—*Steven T. Wright, MD*
Otolaryngology, Head and Neck Surgery
Founder and President, Born to Live Men's Ministry
College Station, TX

INTRODUCTION

Most, if not all of us, are confronted with obstacles, roadblocks, or detours we did not expect at some point in our lives. Some of these can knock the wind out of us and seem overwhelming and insurmountable to overcome when we are face to face with them. These unexpected challenges can be heartrending, thus depleting us physically, emotionally, mentally, financially, relationally, and, yes, even spiritually.

In my personal case, I needed to know the Lord as my Comforter, the Great Physician, and Healer, Provider, Strength, Peace, and Hope in a very trying storm for me and my family when confronted with a diagnosis of 80 percent aggressive B-cell lymphoma cancer. Everyone's story may be different, yet regardless of our personal circumstances, we can fix our eyes on the Author and Finisher of our faith, to know from whence our hope comes.

Little did I realize at the time just how the diagnosis would also affect my family, friends, and many who were following our battle, in different ways. As you read this book, *God Did Not Do This to Me*, by Lisa Stringer, my wife, you will see how after receiving the gut-wrenching news, I drove to the parking lot of a local grocery chain to be alone and process. I can only imagine how difficult this was for my wife and family, who were having to process without me while waiting for me to come home.

This book is written from my wife's perspective, from having to live through this emotional roller coaster not only as my wife, who was battling for her husband in intercession, but also as the primary caregiver through our family's unexpected battle and journey.

Initially, each time Lisa would read a portion of what she was writing to me, it was difficult for me to hear it. When she finally gave me the full rough manuscript to read, it brought back so many memories and emotions that I just couldn't continue. Lisa has captured so many details, timelines, moments, and honest candor that I know the reader will find them personally relatable.

Those who have read the book have said it brought them to tears, chuckles, laughter, and hope in the midst of their own storms. Regardless of what storm or overwhelming challenges you may face, may you find encouragement, peace, and perspective to carry you through it.

As I mentioned earlier, everybody's story may be different. Your storm may not be our storm. But may you, too, be confident of the amazing, great, and abounding grace of God, our refuge and our strength, an ever-present help in times of trouble.

—*Doug Stringer*
Founder/President
Somebody Cares America
Somebody Cares International

1

IN THE BEGINNING

It was a brisk winter day in March 2015 in Haverhill, Massachusetts. We were ministering there at the invitation of Pastor Marlene Yeo, the director of Somebody Cares New England, a chapter of Somebody Cares America, a ministry my husband founded in 1981. Somebody Cares is a network of organizations and churches impacting communities through prayer initiatives, compassion outreaches, and disaster relief. We also encourage and equip leaders globally and we were in New England to do just that—encourage and equip leaders in the region.

We were excited about the potential snow and enjoying the change in scenery. We live in Houston and anyone who is familiar with the weather there during the winter months knows it can be 75 degrees one day and 50 degrees the next.

Doug and I had returned from a full day of ministry assignments to "the Yeo Hotel." Marlene and her husband, Harry, transformed their basement into beautiful guest quarters, with a living room and full kitchen. It is our preferred place to be when ministering in the region.

Doug had settled in a chair at the desk in our cozy room to answer emails on his laptop. Moments later, he turned to me and with a very dismal look and a soft-spoken voice, he said, "I don't feel well; the lump I felt in my throat a few days ago feels larger." I looked at him and stayed quiet for a moment, focusing my eyes on his and then focusing in on his throat, which he kept touching. Sure enough, the lump he had felt on the right side of his throat was now evident.

Perhaps someone who met Doug for the first time would not have noticed the lump, but if you brought attention to it and focused in on his neck, you would see the swelling about the size of a peach pit. We talked about him going to see a doctor upon our return to Houston, and then prayed together, asking God for His healing, grace to continue to serve and not let this be a distraction, and for peace to dwell in both our hearts.

Doug took the initiative to email his cousin, who is a professor and chairman of the Department of Otolaryngology and Communicative Sciences at the University of Mississippi Medical Center. Otolaryngologists are physicians trained in the medical and surgical management and treatment of patients with diseases and disorders of the ear, nose, and throat (ENT). He also emailed a dear friend and partner in ministry, Dr. Steven T. Wright, who after some correspondence, suggested we see an ENT he knows in Houston. He forwarded her information and we were able to get an appointment shortly thereafter.

That day, Doug continued with his responsibilities and spent hours returning emails and studying. Like so many other strong-willed leaders, he didn't allow his mind to be consumed with what wasn't feeling physically right, but focused on his mission and heartfelt assignment.

The next day, after a powerful time of ministry, we returned to the room. It was evident to me that his concern was growing. Often, we put on a strong, public face of great strength, stoically not allowing people to see our emotions.

BOTH THE LUMP AND IMAGINATION GROW

In the privacy of our room, Doug began to let his guard down. He sat back in the chair with an unsettled look on his face. "I think it's getting bigger," he said. Doug grabbed my hand and ran it over the area. It was incredible and disturbing how quickly the lump was visibly growing in size. Moreover, I could see the consternation in Doug's eyes.

> THE MIND, WHEN NOT BROUGHT UNDER THE AUTHORITY OF GOD, CAN NEGATIVELY AFFECT YOUR HEART AND BODY. YOUR WILD IMAGINATION CAN CAUSE UNDUE STRESS.

His concern was my concern multiplied by my mind going into overdrive. The mind, when not brought under the authority of God, can negatively affect your heart and body. Your wild imagination can cause undue stress, which also affects the way the body operates. Second Corinthians 10:5 urges us to "[cast] *down arguments and every high thing that exalts itself against the knowledge of God, bringing every thought into captivity to the obedience of Christ.*"

Never did the thought of cancer come to mind in my moments of processing, *What could this be?* I had been intentional about praying that cancer would never come to any member of my family…because it had taken my father's life. Can you relate to that? There is power in our words and because I was faithful to pray that specifically, then in my mind, it wasn't even a possibility. I didn't know what this abnormal lump was, but I knew a doctor could fix it and, moreover, the doctor of all doctors, Jehovah Rapha, would take care of Douglas, heal him, and make all things work out.

Days earlier, Doug had mentioned to me that something wasn't right. He felt fatigued and sluggish. In fact, he mentioned an awkward feeling in his throat. In retrospect, I realize Doug looked more tired at the end of his long days, but I chalked it up to the stress of the burdens he was carrying. I also recall him touching his throat, stroking it from his neck upwards, much like when he shaves. As I have pondered and processed many memories, I remember Doug stroking his throat at the dinner table, in the car while at a red light, and even lying in bed. Doug is not one to complain. In fact, when he doesn't feel at his best, he is the first to adjust his daily diet by adding natural or organic remedies.

While in New England, we participated in the food pantry distribution to those in need in Haverhill, taped a local television program with Pastor Marlene, and then ministered at the School of Transformation at Citywide Church of greater Lowell. It was there that Doug shared at a bilingual service, which I interpreted in Spanish for those in attendance, who appreciated and needed the translation. Many pastors and leaders from across the region were present. Doug reminded us that we need courageous and persevering leaders for the days in which we lived.

PRAYER BRINGS BREAKTHROUGH

I recall that as the service was coming to a close, Doug had a few words of knowledge for some in attendance. He spoke life over a young man sitting in the congregation, saying he would have a much-needed breakthrough in the next few weeks. After the service, we found out that the young man was a worship leader, husband, and father. His parents are pastors and people of great faith. He had been on a waiting list for years for a kidney transplant and was getting to a very desperate place.

We had no knowledge of that at the time. We left church that day with expectation and continued to pray for this young man daily throughout the following days. Weeks later, we received word that a miracle had taken place: a match was found and he would receive his transplant. Our prayers were now focused on all going well and for his body to welcome the kidney and that it would function as it should. Wesley Hernandez had the surgery and as of the publishing of this book, he continues to flourish and is raising his beautiful family and ministering through song.

Here we were, believing God for a miracle for our new friend and co-laborer, not knowing Doug had cancer growing rapidly in his body. He did not let the discomfort become a distraction that would limit him from doing his kingdom assignment. Doug continued about the Father's business and kept his eyes on the Author and Finisher of our faith.

It was now April 6, the day we were scheduled to see the ear, nose, and throat specialist that Dr. Wright had recommended. With each day that passed, the lump in Doug's throat was getting slightly bigger; every day, I saw him stroking his throat more and more. I don't know that he was aware of how often he was touching his throat. I think it was reactionary to whatever he was feeling in the natural.

April 6 was a much anticipated and very important day for us. We would finally begin the process of getting answers and hopefully a quick fix to whatever was causing the fatigue, discomfort, and now more noticeable lump in his throat. It was also our daughter's thirteenth birthday. Because of our travel schedule and prior commitments, as well as the limited days the doctor had available for new patients, this was the soonest and only day we could see Dr. Deborah Miller.

It was a beautiful morning in early spring. I awoke with joy; after all, this was the day the Lord had made, we were going to get Doug well, and we had a birthday to celebrate. I prepared my husband's coffee to go, gathered my things, loaded the car with what was needed for the day, and awaited for the family to come exiting through the door. We had a joyful thirty-minute ride to the doctor's office. Ashley sang songs like she always does and talked about all the things she wanted to buy during her shopping spree date with her dad.

GPS told us we had arrived. As we unloaded from the car, I could sense that Doug was uneasy. I can only imagine what he was thinking. It was his daughter's birthday and this is not where he wanted to be. He was quiet as we walked toward the elevator and found our way to the office.

The three of us settled in the waiting area and Ashley began to distract us from focusing on the many patients who were waiting to be called back. Her voice was full of excitement as she reminded us of all she wanted to do that day and where we would have her birthday lunch. In the midst of some smiles and laughter, a door opened and a nurse said, "John Stringer, you can come back now." Doug's full name is John Douglas Stringer Jr. He was named after his father and to differentiate between the two, he is known to almost everyone around the globe as Doug Stringer. Ashley and I patiently sat in the waiting room while Doug went back to see the doctor.

WAITING PATIENTLY

Waiting rooms can be a place of reflection, silent prayers, and gratitude for our health, family, and so much more. In the waiting room, you can see many people who, in the natural, look really sick. Some are alone, some are angry, and some fight or argue with each other without any regard for those around them. It amazes me how many use foul language with each other—and how many do it in front of children.

> **IF YOU EVER NEED PERSPECTIVE AND APPRECIATION FOR YOUR OWN HEALTH, GO TO THE WAITING ROOM OF A HOSPITAL OR MEDICAL BUILDING AND YOU WILL SURELY FIND IT THERE.**

If you ever need perspective and appreciation for your own health, go to the waiting room of a hospital or medical building and you will surely find it there within a short window of observation. I tried to entertain Ashley, as I saw her get a bit impatient after a while. In her mind, the doctor would get Daddy healed quickly and we would go on to celebrate her birthday in grand style.

When Doug finally came out into the waiting room, he was quiet, and shared what felt like a simple and courtesy smile. We made our exit to the elevator, where he put Ashley first and began to ask her where she wanted to start her fun day. I, on the other hand, wanted the four-one-one.

After giving Ashley some attention, he shared that the doctor would put him on a ten-day antibiotic, hoping that would work. If it didn't take care of the issue, then they would biopsy one of the lymph nodes. In my mind, the biopsy would not be needed because the antibiotic would take care of whatever infection had made itself present in Doug's body. And besides that, we would pray for his healing and God would answer, just as we had asked of Him.

A DADDY/DAUGHTER TRADITION

Doug focused his attention back on Ashley and off to the mall we went. He has always made it a point to do something extra special for Ashley on her birthday. It was a daddy/daughter tradition. That year, we chose to host a coming-of-age tea with the intercessors who come and pray faithfully for our nation, as well as all the prayer requests we receive from all over the world. To have these seasoned prayer warriors, whom we love dearly and highly esteem, pray over Ashley and speak into her life would be a priceless treasure. The tea would take place many weeks later because of our hectic travel schedule.

First stop was brunch at one of her favorite spots and then we would continue on to the mall for her mini-shopping spree. Doug had taken his laptop with him, so he could sit in a centralized coffee shop in the mall and work while Ashley enjoyed spending her birthday money.

Ashley is the kind of shopper who can spend an hour in each store, carefully studying each piece she may potentially purchase. A deep thinker and visionary, she is very methodical. She enjoys studying the potential of any item she may choose to purchase and often forgets that there is a budget and a time constraint when she walks in. She is all about style and colors—and she loves jewelry. She could shop every other day.

I'm the exact opposite, and so is Doug. I go into a store with a particular purchase in mind. I rarely let other items distract me. I am laughing as I write this because this is a gift. I have told my husband many times how fortunate he is to have me. :) He doesn't have to worry about my overspending on myself. I hope some of you ladies are laughing right about now. I imagine there are some who feel sorry for me, too.

We told Daddy that we would come and check in after each purchase as Ashley had asked for permission to visit at least three stores. Doug was more than willing to release his girls and wait patiently. I imagine that many men can relate as they accompany their wives or children on a shopping mission.

Family time is important to Doug and he's very intentional about making sure Ashley has times of his undivided attention. He also includes her as much as he can in ministry opportunities. Many times, he has said that it makes no sense to help to save others if he is going to lose his own family. Thus, Doug and Ashley have a very special bond. In some ways, they are two peas in a pod because they are both very witty, often playing jokes on me—and sometimes on each other or other people—and both living life with pure joy, looking to seek the good and not the bad in others.

PRAYING FOR GOD'S HEALING FIRST

Our final stop on Ashley's birthday was the pharmacy to pick up the prescription Doug had received that morning. Doug and I prayed over the medicine and asked the Lord to allow it to do only what it was intended to do, with no adverse reaction or side effects. Think of all the commercials for medications on TV that give you hope for a medical issue you might have, but then the voiceover rapidly tells you, "May cause heart attacks or sudden death," and any number of unwanted problems.

Doug has always asked us to pray and ask the Lord for healing before we take anything, giving Him all authority over our lives. I recall the first time he saw me take two Advil out of the bottle and asked what I was doing. I told him I had really bad stomach cramps and needed pain relief so I could continue on our assignments with ease instead of discomfort. He asked me, "Did you pray and ask God to heal you first?" I remember looking at him with disbelief. Of course, I had asked God to take away the pain—I had asked Him as soon as it started.

Sometimes, I share this story with ladies with a big smile on my face, as I know they fully understand my wanting quick relief from pain. In all seriousness, though, I absolutely understand what my husband was trying to teach me. With the advancement of medicine and all that is readily available to many people, we are used to taking pills or medications that will cure or help just about any issue that's not life-threatening. Many don't give it a second thought.

The reality is that as a believer in Christ, we are taught to pray and invite Him to be our Healer, Liberator, and Deliverer:

> *Is anyone among you suffering? Let him pray. Is anyone cheerful? Let him sing psalms. Is anyone among you sick? Let him call for the elders of the church, and let them pray over him, anointing him with oil in the name of the Lord. And the prayer of faith will save the sick, and the Lord will raise him up. And if he has committed sins, he will be forgiven. Confess your trespasses to one another, and pray for one another, that you may be healed. The effective, fervent prayer of a righteous man avails much.*
>
> (James 5:13–16)

I have honored my husband's request to pray before I take anything and feel great peace about including Him even in the littlest of things. I also believe there is honor in honoring my husband's simple yet faith-driven request.

CALLS TO PRAYER

April 8 is our wedding anniversary. Since our return from New England, Doug had traveled to Waco, Texas, to be a part of The Gathering Waco at Baylor University and was fully engaged in working on The Response South Carolina, a call to prayer for a nation in crisis. The latter would take place June 13 and would be a true Joel 2 and 2 Chronicles 7:14 prayer gathering called by then-Governor Nikki Haley. In Joel 2, the prophet declares the day of the Lord, there is a call to repentance, the land is refreshed, and the Holy Spirit is poured out. In 2 Chronicles 7:14, God tells King Solomon, *"If My people who are called by My name will humble themselves, and pray and seek My face, and turn from their wicked ways, then I will hear from heaven, and will forgive their sin and heal their land."*

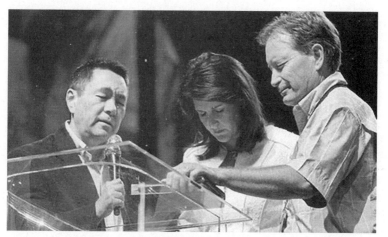

Doug, at left, prays over then-Gov. Nikki Haley of South Carolina with her pastor, Rev. Jeff Kersey of Mt. Horeb United Methodist Church in Lexington.

Facilitating this gathering required many trips to meet with pastors and leaders in the community and share the heart and vision that the Lord had given David and Cindy Lane from the American Renewal Project. It was about churches uniting and awakening so that we could impact the soul of our nation. This was a chance for us to respond corporately and respond in humility, repentance, and renewed consecration, seeking heaven for God's intervention. Doug and the team believed that God could awaken His church and do a work in us and through us so we could impact the soul of our nation in a good way and we could be a blessing to the nations of the world. There was excitement in the air and hope amidst all the negative rhetoric we would receive from the news throughout our nation and around the globe.

A BEAUTIFUL MESSAGE FROM MY HUSBAND

I awoke on the morning of our anniversary with joy and gratitude for the new day, and the fact that my husband left cards on my night stand, knowing they would be the first thing I would see upon getting out of bed. When I signed on to social media I found this beautiful message on my Facebook page:

> Lisa, it's now after midnight and you are asleep. But, as we enter into Wednesday, April 8th, I wanted to say Happy Anniversary! I'm a blessed man to have such a loving family. I always love to come home. As Dorothy in the Wizard of Oz used to say, "There's no place like home!" I love the way you and Ashley, and of course our puppy Asia, always get excited when I arrive home from the office or from a ministry trip. I love our daughter always filling the house with singing and dancing in the Lord. I love our family times together...and so much more. You really are a great wife, mother to our daughter, a daughter to your mother, and a friend to others. We have laughed much, wept over our city, nation and nations...dreamed and believed for the emerging generation, as well as our ministry stewardship. I love the

way you believe in Christ in me, and understanding the burdens I carry in the depths of my heart and soul. I pray I will always bring you the joy, peace and hope that you deserve. I also love the fact that we get to celebrate our anniversary twice a year. Our official intimate wedding on April 8th, as well as our public celebration with many friends and family at the end of May. Anyway, when you wake up and when you read your FB Page, I will have already told you Happy Anniversary, and you will have read the cards I left around, but wanted to keep on letting you know that I love you and it really is a Happy Anniversary! OK, can I have a cappuccino now?

Doug is a big romantic at heart. He loves quality time and has the gift of giving. He is the type of man who will go to a Hallmark store and read through many cards before deciding which is the right one. More often than not, he likes the messages of many of them and will proceed to purchase them all. I have found that outside of him purchasing a gift for me, it is best that I go with him as he will buy the store. As I reflect now on what we did not know prior to receiving the diagnosis, I thank God that my husband was and is intentional about making memories with not just his family but his friends, too. Doug lives in the now and feels strongly about not putting off for tomorrow what you can do today.

As the ten days of taking the antibiotics continued, so did our full schedule. Doug and I noticed that the nodule on his neck was now larger in size and there was no obvious healing taking place. He could feel the disturbance of the increase in size of his node. He felt more fatigued and was just not the full of energy husband and father I was used to seeing. Something was just off.

He reported back to the doctor and she suggested he take the next step of having the nodule biopsied. We would have to find a window to get this outpatient surgery done. Because his assignments are not confined to one city, this would be no easy task. Finding a day that was open for him as well as the hospital would be a challenge. The medical team shared how he would be awake when they inserted a very long needle in his neck to get what was needed for the testing.

It is at times like this that we often realize how much we hurt when our loved ones hurt. As a parent, a spouse, or a best friend, one often wishes we could take the pain for them. I didn't like the fact that my husband would have to endure this procedure; it was not something one naturally wants to do. I saw concern in his face and a desire with all his heart to be an example of strength for Ashley and me.

I recall sitting in the waiting area, praying for peace in his heart and health in his body. I also found myself praying for the many who were in the waiting area, as the stress that some were carrying was quite evident. After the procedure, Doug and I went to a favorite breakfast spot prior to his returning to work. He had been fasting as instructed and had worked up an appetite.

Doug felt the discomfort in his throat was becoming more tangible with every meal, but he would just briefly mention this in our conversations. Days later, we would receive a call that they did not get what they needed and he would have to endure the procedure again. The soonest we could get the second biopsy done was Wednesday, May 6.

From the days of taking the antibiotic and over the next few weeks, we would travel throughout Texas, Boston, New Hampshire, Chicago, Orlando, Atlanta, Alabama, and more.

We had been a part of the National Day of Prayer gathering in Houston, Nights to Honor Israel, and ministry celebrations, and helped to raise funds for the earthquake that had taken place in Nepal, as well as mobilizing help and resources for those affected by it. Ashley was writing and recording music and keeping busy with her schoolwork, extracurricular activities, and volunteer work at the church. We are a family of faith and we kept on doing what we were called to do, praying and believing for Doug's healing...yet wondering how God was going to make all things good for us.

A LIFE-CHANGING PHONE CALL

It was now Friday, May 8, a month since our anniversary and the day that Doug received a phone call that would forever change our lives.

Doug had been part of a live taping at the TBN Houston studios for their telethon week. It was a powerful time of ministry. That afternoon, I recall posting a photo on social media of Doug and the other pastors agreeing in prayer for the needs of the many who called in their requests. With the intensity of rush-hour traffic in Houston, Doug felt his time would be better spent working the remainder of the day at the house rather than spending about two additional hours in traffic to work out of the office for one hour. Doug was in his home office, sipping a cup of coffee, his attention fully on his computer screen. I was in the kitchen preparing a meal and doing some chores.

Doug's cell phone rang and he answered it as he stepped out of the office area. For some reason, his phone service was not that great in our home, so he often had to head outside or sit in his car to take a call or complete it. As he passed me, he said, "Yes, doctor." That got my attention. *Could it be that the doctor was calling with the results?* Doctors usually don't do that; instead, a nurse or someone from the office staff calls. Nonetheless, I was determined to tether myself to him to find out what was going on. You can imagine that with every day that passed, we were in need of relief from this uncomfortable distraction, in need of answers. *What was growing in his neck—and why?*

I was only a few yards behind him. He was already sitting in his car and I didn't ask permission to get in; I just opened the door and sat in the passenger's seat. I proceeded to shut the door as quietly as I could and sat silently, paying attention to every word he said, trying to read his body language. I would look away for a few seconds at a time, trying not to make him more uncomfortable than he already was. After all, he was not given a chance to take the call alone.

"HOW BAD IS IT?"

Doug continued to listen to whatever the doctor was telling him. I could tell something wasn't right because Doug's countenance had changed. It was obvious he was not receiving good news. Whatever it was, at no time did I ever imagine it to be cancer. Doug would not look at me; his eyes were locked in a forward gaze. That alone had my heart beating a tad faster.

I then heard him say, "How bad is it?" Oh, my goodness, was my heart beating right out of my chest! *How bad is it? How bad is what? This can't be bad! I was not expecting bad!* Then I heard the heart-wrenching, horrible "c" word come out of my husband's mouth. He still had his eyes fixed forward. That in itself was painful, not because he wasn't acknowledging me, but because he was hurting and I knew that if we made eye contact, one or both of us would break down at this point.

We had been on an emotional rollercoaster and we were about to take a drop from one of the scariest peaks on one of the worst rides people can experience. I was struggling with everything in me to not allow tears to stream down my face. After all, I was still only hearing one side of the conversation. I recall Doug getting choked up and his voice cracking as he fought back the natural reaction to bad news. He then asked, "What kind of cancer is it?" My heart stopped. I felt like I had been shot and life was moving in slow motion. I could feel every nerve in my body. A deep pain set in.

"Assumption is the lowest form of knowledge" is something my husband learned from Dr. Ed Cole. Doug often says this in our home—and so does Ashley. Sitting in the car, hearing the word "cancer" come out of Doug's mouth, there wasn't much to assume. It's a word no one wants to hear, not because you're afraid of it, but because getting rid of it usually comes at a high cost—physically, emotionally, financially, and in every other way imaginable. And let's face it, many are terrified of the word and its potential consequences, including death.

Doug finished his call with the ENT doctor and continued to stare ahead. He took a deep breath. "It's cancer," he said with a broken voice. His eyes, still fixed ahead, not looking at me, became glossy with tears. He took another deep breath.

"I have large B-cell lymphoma and it's 80 percent aggressive," he told me. "They don't know how bad as they need to run more tests."

I was speechless; all I could do was reach out to touch his hands, which were fixed on the steering wheel. I tried to hold back the tears, but it was a losing battle. I took a deep breath and brushed my cheek against my shoulder, trying to hide the natural effect of my broken heart. I recognize that Doug probably knew this was hard for me to hear, but in the moment, we often try to be emotionally or physically strong for those we love. He tried hard to maintain his composure and did so to the best of his ability as he continued to share more information.

"They have made phone calls and are setting up an appointment to see a doctor at MD Anderson first thing next week," he said. "In fact, I believe they are trying to get us an appointment for Tuesday."

DOUG SPENDS THE DAY ALONE IN PRAYER

Finally, he turned to me. With tears in his eyes and a very choked-up voice, he said, "You go inside. I need to be alone for a while." I didn't want to leave him. I wanted desperately to wrap my arms around him and hug him ever so tightly. I wanted to believe this was just all a bad dream. We gazed at each other for what seemed like an eternity, saying so much with our eyes without even saying a word. In reality, it was probably only a few seconds. He looked away again and said, "I'll be okay. I just need to be alone."

With deep breaths and slow-flowing tears running down my burning cheeks, I nodded with affirmation and acceptance of his desires. "I love you," I told him. I looked away, made my way out of the car, and slowly shut the door. I glanced at him but he only continued to look forward. Then he put the car in reverse and drove away.

I was broken. I felt like I had been painfully punched and my knees were about to buckle. A mammoth weight had just been placed on my shoulders.

2

IT IS WELL WITH MY SOUL

The car was no longer in sight and I proceeded to make my way into our home through the garage. I remember going to my bedroom and shutting the door. I'm not sure to what extent it had all sunk in yet; twenty minutes ago, things were so different. Family life was going on, ministry was taking place as Doug was responding to emails and on calls in his home office, then suddenly with the news from a phone call, my world was turned upside down.

I went to my knees at the foot of Doug's recliner chair, and with tears streaming down my face, I cried out to the Lord. "Please God, protect my husband, mend his hurting heart, and comfort him in his time of need. You are the one true living God who speaks to Your people. Give him strength, God. Your Word says that You never give us more than we can handle— and God, without You, I don't think we can handle this. I need

You in a way I have never needed You before. Take my hand and guide me through the valley of the shadow of death. God, Doug is hurting now and I don't want him to hurt. I'm hurting and I need You to know that I don't understand why You let this happen…but I'm going to trust You. I am not mad at You, but I don't understand right now. I do know this: we have trusted You in the past and we are going to trust You now."

In the midst of my talk with God, I was going through my fair share of tissues as tears continued to stream down my face. Also, at some point in the midst of my petitions to the Lord, I shifted my prayers to declarations over Doug and our family. For the next several minutes, I put on the armor of God and the warrior princess spirit in me came alive.

"YOU SHALL LIVE AND NOT DIE!"

I picked up one of the many Bibles that Doug keeps on his lampstand and I began to raise the sword of the Spirit with authority, declaring His word over Douglas. I remember saying with a loud voice, "Douglas, you shall live and not die!" I paced the floor and continued to read the Scripture out loud and added our names wherever appropriate, making it personal to our family and circumstance. Exodus 23:25 says, "*You shall serve the Lord your God, and He will bless your bread and your water. And I will take sickness away from the midst of you.*" I read it as, "We will worship the Lord our God, and His blessing will be on our food and water. He will take away sickness from among us."

I continued on until my spirit fully believed what I was declaring and peace came upon me. I ended my declarations with Psalm 23:

> *The Lord is my shepherd; I shall not want. He makes me to lie down in green pastures; He leads me beside the*

still waters. He restores my soul; He leads me in the paths of righteousness for His name's sake. Yea, though I walk through the valley of the shadow of death, I will fear no evil; for You are with me; Your rod and Your staff, they comfort me. You prepare a table before me in the presence of my enemies; You anoint my head with oil; my cup runs over. Surely goodness and mercy shall follow me all the days of my life; and I will dwell in the house of the LORD forever.

There is something about reading Psalm 23 and trusting He is able to do what it says. To experience the peace that comes from the words penned by King David, one must truly trust. I have heard Doug mention many a time that we are all given a measure of faith. (See Luke 17:6.) The question is not whether we have faith, as the Bible clearly states that we are all given a measure of it. The question is whether we trust God to do what He says He will do. Trust makes all the difference. I was choosing to trust God and was now resting in a peace that I had not fully experienced in the past hour of my life. I was feeling much better as I was no longer feeling the full weight of what I was carrying. I had released it to the Lord.

> THE BIBLE CLEARLY SAYS WE ARE ALL GIVEN A MEASURE OF FAITH. THE QUESTION IS WHETHER WE TRUST GOD TO DO WHAT HE SAYS HE WILL DO.

I walked over to Doug's recliner and as I slowly sat back and took in a few deep breaths, I glanced at my watch and realized Doug had been gone for close to an hour at this point. Tears began to stream down my eyes once more, as I envisioned him alone. I too felt alone, but I was home with the family I had yet to tell.

Not knowing what was going through Doug's mind or how long he would truly be gone, I chose to go upstairs and share the news with both Ashley and my mom, who lives with us. Questions began to bombard my mind. *What would I say? How would I tell them? Together or separately?* I needed to keep my composure, to be strong for them.

I didn't have any details, all I knew is that we were in an unexpected battle that would surely cause change in our home and the ministry we steward. *Am I doing the right thing by telling them? Or should I wait until Doug returns?* If I tell them myself, this would give them time to let the news settle in, and for each of them to have their own intimate time of reflection with the Lord, the way I did. I wanted Doug to return home and not feel the pressure of having to share this with his daughter or mother-in-love. He had enough to think about already and I am sure his mind, like mine, was racing with thoughts. I wanted him to sense peace in our home, not a lack of trust in God. I wanted him to sense that we believed that all would be okay. The choice was made, I would tell them what little I knew.

MY DAUGHTER, MY PRAYER PARTNER

I determined to tell Ashley first. As I took each step toward the staircase and made my way to her room, I was still not sure exactly what I would say. I think in part I was numb, if you can imagine that. Ashley has been my prayer partner since she was three years old. I would get her up at the crack of dawn and we would worship the Lord together without time constraint. After we sensed peace and His presence, we would pray for our needs, our friends, the nation, the military, peace in Israel, and so much more. It was something we did daily for years. We saw God move mightily in the lives of many we interceded for as well as our own lives. Praying was what we did, and intercession was and is a big part of who we are.

I found Ashley in her room working on her curriculum. She has been homeschooled since the third grade and our schedule varied from week to week, depending on our ministry and family assignments. Some days we work more in the mornings and other days we work into the evening. I recall sitting on the sofa in her room and asking her to stop what she was doing as we needed to have an important talk.

Ashley is a very sensitive young girl, discerning the emotional state of those around her. She must have noticed the expressions on my face or the fact that my eyes were probably a tad swollen from the tears. My nose too must have been a bit red from all the wiping because she sat next to me and gave me a hug. She nestled into my chest and told me, "Whatever it is, Mommy, it's going to be okay."

I began to share the little we knew. "Ashley, you know the lump in Daddy's throat?" She stared intently at me; our eyes were locked in each other's. "The doctor called us today and told Daddy what is causing the swelling." The tears that I had been fighting back began to stream down my face ever so slowly, I could hardly talk. I took a deep breath and said, "The doctor says that Daddy has cancer."

I would like to tell you I kept my composure and that I was a pillar of strength for our little girl, but I would be lying. Tears now streamed down my face at an uncontrollable rate. I then said, "Ashley, we need to pray!" She immediately hung her head down and would not look at me. Not a tear in her eyes, nor a look of fear in her face. She was more stoic in her gaze forward. I then told her, "There is nothing impossible for God. I don't understand why we are facing this, but I know that God will see us through. This is a very serious situation and we need to fervently pray without ceasing. We need to fight for Daddy's life in prayer and intercession."

Ashley internalizes her emotions. She puts up a strong front, but inside, she can carry the hurt deeply. I reminded her how much we loved her, and again how we were going to get through this. Still no tears flowed down her face. I knew she understood what it meant for someone to be diagnosed with cancer. She knew that it had been the cause of death for my father many years before she was born. She had also accompanied Doug and me on many hospital visits to pray for people who were battling cancer. MD Anderson Cancer Center in Houston, as well as other hospitals and hospice facilities, were not unknown to her. I believe she understood that the news was not good. Ashley was probably not expecting her father to be in a battle that she had seen so many others fight. Truthfully, I wasn't expecting this type of health battle either.

Ashley had nothing to say to me. I asked her how she felt and if she had any questions. I got nothing out of her but a nod. She was silent. I scooted over to her and gave her a big hug, reminding her again how much we loved her. She was limp and did not hug me back. Ashley was lost in thought and knowing her, she put up a wall to block out any chance of letting me see her cry. She wanted to be strong for me, for us, and that was okay. Everyone processes differently, and I needed to give her the grace and space to do so. With that, I turned away and walked out of her room.

REALITY SINKS IN

I went into the guest bedroom we had upstairs and muffled my cry with a pillow. *What just happened? What is happening?* The control and peace I had found downstairs in my time with God was not what I was demonstrating at this time. I guess the reality of the pain of what was taking place was hitting me like a flood. I cried for a few more seconds and then took another deep breath, wiped away more tears, cleared my nose, and asked God for grace to share the news with my mother. "I can do this," I told myself. "You are my strength, Lord." I would declare this over and over until no more tears flowed from my eyes.

My parents were married forty-one years. They loved each other and were going to be together forever. My dad was diagnosed with pancreatic cancer and given six months to live. He lived four of those months before graduating to his eternal home in heaven. The effects of the cancer destroying my dad's body were heartbreaking. My mom saw how much dad was challenged and the amount of pain he was in, and that left in her an ingrained negative association with the word *cancer*. Not that cancer isn't negative for everyone, it's just that some are able to overcome it without some of the horrible side effects. Others catch the disease at an early stage and deal with it before it turns their world upside down and their bodies into an unfortunate battlefield.

I had regained my composure and taking more deep breaths, I remember asking myself, "How on earth am I going to tell her?" This would bring back a flood of unfavorable memories for her. I made my way down the hall and walked into her room. She was sitting on her bed watching a news program. "Mami..." I began, which is what we call my mom in Spanish. Then I broke down. I could not even speak. Tears began to stream down my face like a great flood. She, of course, became startled and asked, "What is it? What's wrong? What happened?" I began to tell her that Doug received a call from his doctor and they determined that he had cancer. She yelled out, "No! No! This can't be." She began to cry loudly and said, "I'm so sorry, honey, I'm so sorry." I told her, "I'm sorry, too." I gave her a big hug and grabbed tissues for both of us. My heart was overwhelmed for her, as she loves Doug very much, and our immediate family consists of all four of us, grandma included. I knew instantly that I could relate to her in a way I never had before. I told her, "Mami, pray, just pray."

She wanted to know where Doug was. I told her he needed to be alone, to spend time talking with God. She looked down, tears running down her face, but couldn't speak. She tried to speak, but she couldn't. She was hurting and it was evident. I told her I loved her and that we would all be okay. She just nodded her head as she fiddled with the tissue in her hands. "Doug will overcome this." I affirmed, "We all will, because God is in control." I left her alone so she could have her own moments of reflection, prayer, and time with the Lord.

It was done, everyone in our home now knew.

ASHLEY STAYS IN HER PRAYER CLOSET

After leaving mom's room, I walked over to check on Ashley, but she wasn't in her room. I checked in her bathroom and proceeded to go into every room upstairs. *Where could she be?* I then went downstairs, checking every room there. She was nowhere to be found. At this point, my heart was pounding and my knees were weak once more. After not finding her in several other places around the house, I was desperate and concerned. *Where did she go?*

I finally opened the door to her closet and there she was, curled in the fetal position, lying on the floor. Her cell phone was near her ear playing worship music ever so softly. I could breathe with ease and my heart could begin to beat at a normal rate. I fell to my knees to comfort her as I realized at that moment how deeply she was hurt as she processed what was happening to Daddy. I asked, "Are you okay?" She immediately said, "Please leave, I want to be alone." My heart was broken for her and there wasn't much I could do. I tried engaging her but realized it wasn't the time.

I guess all of us needed our moments to grieve and reflect. We needed to process our thoughts, to pray and talk to God, and in the midst of it all, cry and release the confusion and disappointment. We were about to embark on an unexpected journey that we didn't fully understand. We all knew the process could and likely would be painful, but not fighting to the best of our ability was not an option for any of us. We had to trust God for His promises to our family that were yet to be fulfilled, choose to have hope, and cling to the hand of God as tightly as we could. We would fight with everything we had and, in the end, we were determined to trust God, no matter what the outcome was.

Hours went by before Doug would call to check in. I remember the call like it was yesterday: "Hi, I'm just calling to let you know I'm okay." There was silence for a few seconds. "I've been at a grocery parking lot. I needed time with God and to process." You can imagine that his voice sounded a bit weak and tired, or perhaps it was the voice of someone who had just experienced disappointment. "Did you tell mom and Ashley?"

"Yes," I responded with a gentle voice.

"How are they doing?" He let me know that he was on his way home and wanted to have a family meeting, requesting that I have communion elements ready.

DOUG MAKES A BIG ANNOUNCEMENT

The four of us gathered in the family room, everyone rather quiet, emotionally exhausted, and with runny noses and tissues in hand.

Doug told about his time with God and wanted to share what he was confident of. "God did not do this to me—and if He did not do this to me, then it doesn't belong to me!"

Wow! I had to let that sink in for a moment. Yes, that is what I needed to hear. God didn't do this.

Doug had his armor of God on and it was evident the warrior spirit in him was speaking. He was broken, but he was all in for the battle before us and was determined to not retreat in fear. He continued, "If it doesn't belong to me then it's not going to be about me. We are going to turn this into intercession for our country." That took a moment to sink in: we would turn this into a time of intercession for our nation. It made sense. I could do that—*we* could do that!

It was a presidential election year and political rhetoric dominated the news almost every day. It felt like we were a divided nation at the time, and it was even evident in churches and among the people in the pews. What we needed was people praying and praying was what we did personally, as a family, and corporately.

To end our time together, Doug led our family in prayer. We encouraged each other a bit (mostly, he encouraged us) and then we took communion as a family, acknowledging complete dependence on the great I Am. We had also determined to take communion together every day or, at the least, until this trial was over. We sat in silence for a while and one at a time, each of us went quietly our own direction.

After a short while had passed, I went to ask Doug some important questions that needed to be addressed, like who do we share the news with? When? We resolved that we needed to inform our friends and ask for their prayers. Doug has taught us that relationships define our destiny, first with God, and then with one another. He has ministered and sown seed around the globe for decades and has been blessed to keep long-lasting relationships on every continent.

We determined that this was not something we could or should keep to ourselves. Our friends and spiritual family would want to know. Psalm 145:18 reminds us, *"The LORD is near to all who call upon Him."* This was a time we needed and wanted the prayers of all who were willing to call upon the Lord and lift Doug and our family up before the throne of God.

DETERMINED TO PRESS ON

I offered to write the letter that we would post on social media. Then Doug and Dr. Jodie Chiricosta, vice president of Somebody Cares International, could use it as a base to develop a more specific letter to the ministry board members and partners. We talked about what this could mean to our ministry schedule and both determined that no matter what, if this was a spiritual attack, then we would not allow our commitment to The Response South Carolina, a prayer gathering that was coming up in June, to be interrupted. Nor would we allow this to interrupt what we felt were the assignments God had given us to serve our city and nation.

> THERE IS POWER IN PRAYER, AND THE LAST THING THE ENEMY WANTS TO SEE IS PEOPLE GATHERING IN REPENTANCE AND INTERCESSION BEFORE THE KING OF KINGS.

We would wait on future meetings with the oncologist before we would determine what to do about our international commitments. So without giving it a second thought, we would press forth to see that the Joel 2 gathering would take place in South Carolina, and we would give it our all. There is power in prayer, and the last thing the enemy wants to see is people gathering in repentance and intercession before the King of Kings. Mountains can be moved and the atmosphere changed when His people pray. In fact, we believe our gathering was providential. I'll share more in a later chapter.

The following is what we agreed to share and what I posted on social media and sent via email to friends and ministry leaders on May 8, 2015:

> Seven weeks ago Doug noticed some discomfort in his throat. Today we received word that he has lymphoma cancer. The extent to which it has spread to his body is yet to be determined. We will learn more this coming week as we begin seeing doctors at MD Anderson.
>
> After a few hours of processing, Doug wrote a letter to his board members and some advisors. I would like to share part of what he wrote: "As my friend, Tan Sri Dr. Francis Yeoh, has often reminded us through his love for Horatio Spafford's song, 'It Is Well with My Soul.' Yes, I have great peace and it is well with my soul. Thank you very much for your love and prayers. As I have learned from my friends Robert and Karyn Barriger in Peru, I do not need to leave my calling for my healing, for my healing is in my calling. In Him I live, move, and have my being. It is an honor to serve the Lord and His people."
>
> We have already been inundated with many loving calls and texts. We apologize for the impersonal way of sharing this but felt this would be an easier way to communicate to some of you, as we journey in the victory through the Lord. As Doug always says, "God always leads us in triumph through Christ Jesus." As a side

note, he seems to be living out his message, "Our desire to win must be greater than our moments of challenge," once more. I could have done without this challenge, but God will see us through.

Doug has prayed for people for thirty-four years in their time of need and healing. Isaiah 58 says that in our time of need, our healing will come speedily. We hold on to the promises of God.

Our love to you,
The Stringer family

MESSAGES OF LOVE, PRAYERS POUR IN

After posting the message on social media, the number of texts and calls that began to come in multiplied greatly. We were without words at the love and expression that was being shared with us. Our world as we knew it had changed in a matter of hours, and I must admit that it was a bit overwhelming. Doug never left his desk. He worked, prayed, pondered, read, and responded to some of the messages. I gave him his privacy, and truthfully, I needed my space as well. I recall going to my study in our home and reading some of the responses to my post.

Tears began to stream down my face; at times so many that I could not see the text in front of me. I chose to turn off the social media sites; although there were many words of life, encouragement, prayers, and hope shared, my heart at that time was too sensitive to not react without the flood of tears streaming down my face time and again.

I put on worship music, had a long time of prayer, and I simply worshipped the Lord. I needed to articulate to the Lord what He already knew, that I would trust Him for Doug's healing, and that I didn't understand His plan, and perhaps I didn't even like it, but I would stay as close to Him as possible. I made a commitment to take care of His precious son and servant, Douglas, and I would be a pillar of strength for our family. I needed to tell Him how much I was hurting, not that He didn't already know. I just needed to spend intimate time crying on my Abba Father's shoulder and declaring my love for Him no matter what.

The next morning, I posted a note on social media. I needed to take the time to express our love and gratitude for all the encouragement, expressions of love, and prayers that were poured out upon us. I had taken the time to read through most of the comments and encouraging Scriptures posted. We were more than blessed. I mentioned that tears were streaming down my face as I read many of the notes, but they were tears of gratitude for His amazing love shown to us through His people, our friends. I was without adequate words that could express the depth of our gratefulness for each person and prayer. The post also closed with this: "May this journey which we have embarked on be quick, full of His grace, provision in every way, and most of all, may it bring Him the glory due His name. God is more than able to meet each and every one of our needs, and I don't mean ours personally, I mean all of us who are in need and believe. We trust the Lord with all that concerns us."

With every post came more support and words of life. It was posts like the ones below from people we love, respect, and honor that stimulated and propelled us forward with courage and faith that moves mountains.

Dr. Karen Kossie-Chernyshev wrote the following:

Lisa, God is with you and Doug, as you already know. You have begun to experience a depth of love and compassion from others that you could not have truly known without the trial you are facing. For years, you have demonstrated and encouraged others to show that "somebody cares." You have loved on God's people selflessly and profusely. Now, God, in His divine wisdom and way, is allowing us to individually and collectively express our love for you and all you continue to mean to us! I am praying for you daily. Love, Karen Kossie-Chernyshev

Dr. Buddy Hicks wrote:

In early 1970, I was diagnosed with a life-threatening vein disease. I had gone in for an examination for a possible minor surgery. The doctor immediately checked me in to the hospital to do exploratory surgery the next morning. As I lay in bed that night in the hospital, I prayed, "Lord, we have a problem. I would not change one day I have lived with and for you. I just want you to know that I will continue to pursue your heart and stay steady in the ministry that you have called me to." I went sound to sleep. The next morning, following the surgeon's exploratory work, he came to visit me after I awoke. He said to me, "I don't know what's going on here. I opened up the area and there is nothing negative there." After the minor surgery, four months later, I was skiing in Colorado. Doug has the same faith and attitude of heart!

Youth Reach Houston Founder Curt Williams wrote, "We are going to war! (In prayer of course.)"

Yes, this was war—and we were determined to win!

3

THIS IS HOW I FIGHT MY BATTLES

It was Tuesday, May 12, exactly eight weeks since our journey had begun. We made our way to the MD Anderson Clear Lake Campus. Doug's ENT made the appointment for us and it wasn't an option to pass on her kind gesture to get him in so quickly. Getting insurance clearance can take a few days and often times there can be a month's wait to see a particular doctor.

Upon checking in, we received our very own patient welcome folder—something we didn't know existed, much less ever wanted to receive.

Doug also received an identification bracelet, much like the ones you receive when you are a patient at a hospital. When they put it around his wrist, another level of reality began to set in. It's as though I immediately had a greater compassion and empathy for those who had the band on and for those who walked with them.

As we waited for the doctor to come into our room, we pondered the many friends we have prayed for at this very hospital, some of whom are doing well and others who are now rejoicing in the presence of God.

Nonetheless, we were strong in the Lord, knowing He was with us every step of the way. We focused our thoughts on the many opportunities we would have to share His love during this journey, and had determined to take one day at a time, never forgetting that He was more than able to heal.

Later that day, Doug posted on my Facebook page, "The Lord is gracious and kind, full of mercy and love. Our God reigns! He is the Great Physician."

Doug was speaking life over himself and encouraging us all along the way, again acknowledging God was Jehovah Rapha, our Healer, and the Doctor of all doctors. If it were not for the Word of God that uplifts, I would have spent most of my time depressed and without authentic hope for healing.

Every day, we were encouraged by different Scriptures; our chosen Scripture for that day was Isaiah 41:10: *"So do not fear, for I am with you; do not be dismayed, for I am your God. I will strengthen you and help you; I will uphold you with my righteous right hand"* (NIV).

"Do not fear!" That is something often easily said, but not always easy to walk in. Even so, I could receive it because God said it and He means it. Our all-knowing and all-powerful God knew that these very words would give me courage in times of weakness. *"I am with you; do not be dismayed."* God is telling us to not be afraid, discouraged, or upset. This did not take Him by surprise.

Essentially, for those of us who choose to trust Him, He is saying, "I am your God. I will strengthen you and help you." I knew God was saying to me, to us, "I've got this. I am more than able. Just don't lose faith."

FAITH FOR HEALING IS POWERFUL

I liken exercising faith for Doug's healing in this season to taking vitamins on a daily basis to get the nutrients one needs to remain healthy. If I were not intentional in reading the Word of God daily and throughout the day, my body, specifically my mind, would become weak. The mind is a powerful tool. I have heard stories of people who were healthy but bought into a lie that they were sick and consequently began to feel ill until they were physically defeated. I recognized the power of words and activating faith.

Proverbs 18:4 (TPT) says, "*Words of wisdom are like a fresh, flowing brook—like deep waters that spring forth from within, bubbling up inside the one with understanding.*" And Proverbs 15:4 (TPT) says, "*When you speak healing words, you offer others fruit from the tree of life. But unhealthy, negative words do nothing but crush their hopes.*"

During this season, I needed hope; I needed the extra vitamins in the natural as my schedule was far from normal and the demand on my time had increased. I also needed the very important spiritual vitamin: extra time in His word to be encouraged and instructed by Him on how to fight this battle. This included additional knee time and greater intimacy with the Lord.

After leaving the doctor's office, we were more determined than ever to keep our focus on our calling and not let the detour become a distraction. We were scheduled to attend a concert in Houston at the Jewish Community Center, celebrating Israel's sixty-seventh anniversary. A friend and Orthodox Jewish rabbi,

Emanuel Zadok, was visiting from Israel and attending the concert. He had heard of the recent diagnosis and asked if he could pray for Doug. Wow, was it powerful as he rebuked any attacks by Satan or ungodly words spoken against him. He then prayed an amazing Abrahamic blessing and spoke prophetically over Doug's life in ways only the Lord or those close to him would know.

We met Rabbi Zadok through a mutual friend during a trip to Israel a few years prior to Doug's diagnosis. The rabbi prays with a confidence that God hears his prayers and is moved into action. Rabbi Zadok would continue to call us from Israel on a regular basis to pray for Doug and get updates on his health. He was always confident that God would heal his friend and that Doug's time on earth was not yet over.

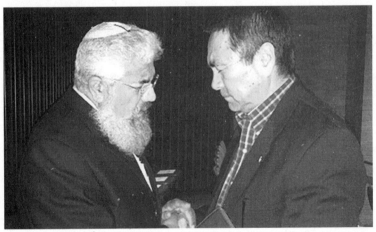

Rabbi Emanuel Zadok prays for Doug after learning about his cancer diagnosis.

One is always grateful for prayers; in fact, in our times of need, we are often more receptive to them. For many of us, it is not that we don't believe healing can come; we just wonder if it can or will come for us. The thought of trusting for big miracles can be a challenge in and of itself.

Too often we hear of seemingly impossible situations become miraculous testimonies for His glory, but fail to embrace that we too can experience them. We believe it can happen for someone else but doubt greatly for ourselves. Many of us feel unworthy of His mercy, touch, and favor, yet the Bible reminds us we are saved *"not because of righteous things we had done, but because of his mercy… [which] he poured out on us generously through Jesus Christ our Savior"* (Titus 3:5–6 NIV).

> TOO OFTEN WE HEAR OF SEEMINGLY IMPOSSIBLE SITUATIONS BECOME MIRACULOUS TESTIMONIES FOR HIS GLORY, BUT FAIL TO EMBRACE THAT WE TOO CAN EXPERIENCE THEM.

In the midst of all Doug was doing for the kingdom, he now had a significant roadblock to deal with. We were determined to not let this be the focus, but instead, as he says, we would reroute, take a detour, and find a way to ultimately arrive at our destination. What was our destination? It was to live out Acts 20:24, to *"finish [our] race with joy, and the ministry which [we] received from the Lord Jesus, to testify to the gospel of the grace of God."* We knew we had assignments and missions to complete. We would not quit, no matter what. That was non-negotiable.

Two mornings later, Doug kept his word, as he was determined to not allow the circumstance or diagnosis to keep him from his assignment and destiny. He departed Houston for a scheduled trip to various cities throughout South Carolina to share about "The Response South Carolina, A Call to Prayer," scheduled to take place on June 13. This was a Joel 2 gathering called for by then-Governor Nikki Haley.

The word of the Lord would continue to go forth from Doug's lips and by his actions. Doug was determined to preach the gospel. He said the Lord knew his appointed time, whether he had a few more days, or decades to live. God knew and he would live his days sharing the good news with a world in need to the best of his ability.

RESEARCHING NATURAL PROTOCOLS

While Doug was away, I dedicated all my free time to researching the specific cancer that he was diagnosed with. I felt like I was becoming an expert in an area that just days before I knew nothing about. My husband trusted me to read up on natural protocols so that he could keep his focus on the assignments before him. We wanted to find and implement protocols to help the body fight off the cancer as organically as possible. The amount of information available via the Internet was absolutely overwhelming as I tried to decipher what was opinion verses fact, and take into consideration what was proven via medical research.

Reading testimonials from people who experienced success with natural remedies was a challenge. When one is emotionally spent, what may otherwise seem like an easy task can blur one's ability to receive without bias. I recall the tears that would stream down my face when I read of the struggles that many encountered. Some lived and some died. Needless to say, my heart was experiencing emotions that would forever transform me.

Let me remind you that at this point, Doug had been diagnosed with lymphoma cancer, but didn't know the extent of it, nor the exact type, and we had yet to have the adequate test done to determine the stage the cancer was considered to be in. We knew the lump on Doug's neck was growing daily and that he was fatigued in the natural. His schedule was intense and I am sure the daily stresses contributed to that.

Some suggested that I stay completely away from the Internet. I will not tell you what I think you should do, other than follow your heart. For some, it can be a means to gather experiences and better understand what you will possibly encounter in your journey. For others, it will be too much to absorb and can be a source of added stress. You will know what to do; just allow His peace to rule over you. *"A joyful heart is good medicine, but a broken spirit dries up the bones"* (Proverbs 17:22 NASB). Don't allow what you read to break or crush you. If it knocks you down, change your reading material, go offline, and pick up His word. Allow Him to help you stand once more.

Shortly after having shared our story via email and social media, we began to hear back from people who followed the ministry we steward, friends, spiritual family from across the globe, and complete strangers who chose to reach out to us. It was impossible to get to all the messages in my email box or those who had private messaged me via social media. People reached out from six of the seven continents. In fact, it took me weeks if not months to respond to some. If for some reason I missed you, please accept my apology. Many of the emails or private messages contained suggestions for treatment, locations of places Doug could be treated both in the U.S. and abroad, and a long list of suggested protocols of every type imaginable.

THE GOOD, THE BAD, AND THE UGLY EMAILS

I must confess that not every email was positive. I will also admit that the timing of some of the emails were either not good, or not what I needed at the time. I have been taught to give grace as I need grace. So know that I am not mad at those who sent emails that seemed harsh at the time, I know everyone meant well and all of us have different means of expressing ourselves. Some of us are just a bit bolder than others.

However, if I am to truly provide insight into our world during this season, I should include the good, the bad, and the ugly. Some of the emails were compassionate, filled with prayers and Scriptures that gave me hope. I took the time to read every one. Perhaps that is why it took so long to respond. God truly used many people to give me a drink of water in a time of need. In fact, they gave my entire household water. When I, as the main caregiver for my husband, was able to be nourished and filled by the written and spoken encouragement, it would flow easily to the family. When caregivers are tired and weak, their actions can reflect the natural need for rest or emotional strain, and the result is impatience and body language that reflects just that. But when their cup is overflowing with love, support, encouragement, and peace, it likewise overflows to those they are caring for. In some emails, if a Scripture was only referenced but not fully noted, I looked it up. I didn't want to miss a bit of what God was saying to me through the many who took the time to write to me or the family. We also used some of the emails that included prayers and Scriptures as devotionals for the family during this season.

Some of the emails, however, were a tad unsympathetic in the way they expressed their opinion and suggested protocol for Doug. I was told by some to stay away from chemotherapy and other pharmaceutical treatments. I can appreciate their good intent and concern, but the way some passionately suggested what we should do or not do only added to the stress I was already feeling and maneuvering through.

> THE WORLD AROUND US GETS CLOUDED AT TIMES AND WE NEED SPIRITUAL CLARITY AND HOLY SPIRIT HEADLIGHTS TO GET US THROUGH THE FOG. —DOUG

I never shared with Doug the emails that burdened me because he did not need to be distracted or give his mind over to internal battles. Doug has said, "The world around us gets clouded at times and we need spiritual clarity and Holy Spirit headlights to get us through the fog." I certainly experienced foggy moments. This is why it is so important to lay it all before the throne of God, to have an intimate relationship with Him so you can hear from Him directly what your path should be, then embrace that path, and trust in Him, no matter what the outcome will be.

I would like to thank those that sent us samples of what natural supplements they suggested. Doug still implements some in his diet as of the publishing of this book. I can never say thank you enough to everyone who emailed, texted, or called, for your patience with me or us, for your unwavering love, grace, financial gifts to cover medical expenses, and so much more. I am even grateful for the few emails that were hard to read. They are all a part of the story that is now a testimony to His abounding grace.

On May 18, I posted the following on Facebook:

The last 24 hours have been a rollercoaster ride of emotions, compounded with a full schedule, a long list of things to do, and a tired body. I found myself a bit emotional, hungry at times but no desire to eat; tears streamed down my face as thoughts raced through my mind. Grateful to God for giving us revelation about certain things and strategy on how to overcome.

I turned on the worship music, woke up Ashley, and asked her to join me in prayer; it was time to go to battle. Tonight, my handsome prince would arrive home from ministry time throughout the state of South Carolina. I wrote a new message on our family board, quoting Psalm 91:1 (ESV): "*He who dwells in the shelter of the Most High will abide in the shadow of the Almighty.*"

PRAYING FOR GOD TO INCREASE HIS GRACE

What a powerful verse! Under His covering is protection—physical, emotional, financial, and spiritual. Our friend Alan Richardson reminded us what evangelist and author Leonard Ravenhill would often preach, that "as Christians, we should not pray for God to lighten the load, but for God to increase His grace for us to bear it." When you receive a word of encouragement from someone who has been through something similar, it is easier to receive from him, for you know he has been tried and tested, and is still able to shine God's light in the midst of the storms. Alan's comment was a perfect reminder that day that we were not to complain about the circumstance, but to continually ask for His grace to get through it.

Doug was only scheduled home for a few days and was to return to MD Anderson, but now to the main campus in the medical center. It is world-renowned and one of the original three comprehensive cancer centers in the United States. To give you an idea how big this hospital is, in 2017, more than 137,000 people sought treatment. Hospital admissions were just under 29,000 and outpatient clinic visits, treatments, and procedures were just under 1.5 million. MDA is completely dedicated to the treatment of those with cancer. So when you walk through its doors, you know everyone with the patient ID bracelet has a common bond.

In his short time home, Doug had a PET scan, CT scan, chest X-rays, blood work, bone marrow biopsies, and more. Doug says, "Passivity causes us to miss God's window of opportunity while the opportunity exists." With this in mind, in every waiting room we sat in, Doug made friends. He engaged people, made some smile, made others laugh, and prayed for all he encountered, whether staff, patient, family, or friend of the patient.

MD Anderson isn't the happiest place on earth, but it is a place where God is ever present. It is also a place of hope for many who are on their journey and for the family members who are believing for their loved one's healing. I compliment the staff, as they are some of the most compassionate and considerate hospital employees we have ever met.

A few days later, I dropped Douglas off at the airport early in the morning. He was scheduled to minister in Seattle, Washington. I was unsure if he would actually go, until I saw him walk away with his luggage; he smiled for me as he walked off and my heart was heavy, yet full of admiration. I prayed he would be strengthened and could only imagine what God had planned over the next few days. He had been feeling a bit achy, and the growth on his neck had increased in size and was getting to be a bit more uncomfortable. We pondered and prayed as whether to honor the commitment or stay home and rest. We laid many prayers before the Lord regarding this trip. In the end, ministering at the Vietnamese conference alongside Pastor Khan Huynh became a reality.

My admiration and love for Doug only grew. We prayed that as he poured out, the Lord would continually pour into him, and we prayed that he would find his healing in his calling.

4

STAGE 4

It was June 4, a day after my birthday. We woke up early, had our individual and family prayer time, did our normal morning routines, and headed to the hospital. This was the day we would get the detailed diagnosis and plan for treatment. I was calm and cool on the outside, but on the inside, I had butterflies. Philippians 4:6–7 says:

> Be anxious for nothing, but in everything by prayer and supplication, with thanksgiving, let your requests be made known to God; and the peace of God, which surpasses all understanding, will guard your hearts and minds through Christ Jesus.

I kept saying this Scripture in my mind over and over again. Anytime my mind would wander and my imagination would take off to unnecessary places, I would repeat the Scripture again.

Doug was making every effort to show us peace, but I sensed the heaviness he was carrying, the physical fatigue he was battling, and the discomfort he had from the growth on his neck. He didn't have to tell me it hurt or bothered him; to me, it was quite obvious as he would occasionally put his hand to his throat and rub it, almost as when he is shaving. When he noticed that I discerned what he was doing, he would give me a quick smile, as though touching his neck was a normal activity and I had nothing to worry about, but he couldn't fool me. I would usually smile back and we would try to move on, neither of us wanting to allow our emotions to get the best of us. We did not want to give too much attention to the negative changes that we were witnessing and he was feeling.

Parking in one of the hospital's massive, multistory garages can be a challenge. Depending on the time of day you arrive, most of the garages are full with exception of the high level floors. Valet parking is also popular at the hospital, but the cost adds up when you are there on a very regular basis. In addition, dropping off your car usually isn't a problem, but I have waited for well over forty minutes to have the car brought back because of the many in need of this service for the ease of loading and unloading a patient with limited mobility.

Anyone who has visited MD Anderson knows the heaviness you feel as soon as you walk in the cancer center. Walk down any given hall or wing of the hospital and you will see patients of every kind—young, old, people from all over the world, of every ethnicity and religious belief.

Some are in good spirits and some look like they have been depleted of every ounce of energy. I will never forget seeing a patient in one of the atriums sitting in his wheelchair underneath a beautiful gazebo. We were walking toward the outpatient chemo waiting area. He was wearing his hospital gown and sitting by himself with a wrap around his head and his IV pole next to him with many drip bags hanging from it.

His eyes were fixed and intently looking forward, as though he was lost in thought, not allowing himself to be distracted by any of the activity around him. It was evident that part of his skull had been removed. *My goodness, what was his story? What would be our story? What will we have to undergo before experiencing the victory we were determined to see? Dare I not feel sorry for myself or the circumstance we found ourselves in?* I took captive my vain imagination and began to intercede for the young man, asking God for his healing and strength to overcome the obstacle before him. I realized ever more that as Doug said the day he was diagnosed with cancer, this wasn't about him, it was about the ministry of presence we now had at one of the best hospitals in the world.

PRAYING FOR OTHER PATIENTS

We were determined to not just walk past every patient on our way to our appointments, but instead we would take the time to stop and pray for those we felt the leading to do so. We would engage patients and caregivers alike, share some smiles, conversations about the Lord, baseball, the weather, and the future. You see, no matter what the outcome, you must believe there is a future, whether on earth or in heaven.

> *"For I know the plans I have for you," declares the* Lord,
> *"plans to prosper you and not to harm you, plans to give you*
> *hope and a future."*   (Jeremiah 29:11 NIV)

Doug often says, "Discouragement is a powerful drug that can distract us from our intended destination, and focusing on our disappointments can lead to disillusionment that will distract us from God's intended destiny for each of us. During these times, it's important to remember that God has a plan and a purpose far greater than the temporary circumstances that plague us."

With this in mind, getting other patients to talk about the future, plans they had, places where they wanted to travel, and things they wanted to experience was a way of seeing many smiles on people's faces who otherwise just sat and stared with glazed eyes or tears.

We made it to the check-in area and settled into an open row of four seats. Doug sat on the end of our row and was focused on filling out some required paperwork prior to being called back. As I looked around the waiting room, I saw men and women who had lost their hair. Some had IV ports sticking out of their arms or protruding from their collar bone area. Some had lost limbs and some were in wheelchairs, too weak to walk. I witnessed family members who were patient with their loved ones, and others that were irritated with the one they were helping or caring for. I saw many who were alone.

Within a few minutes, a lady who had lost her hair had asked if the seat to my left was available. From that moment on, we talked until she was called back. She was in the midst of her battle. Tall, slender, with a beautiful smile, she introduced herself as Karen—and she was a talker, asking what type of cancer Doug had and what stage he was in. I shared that we were there to find out and begin treatment. She began to tell of her experience. Karen said within a very short time of starting chemotherapy, she had lost her hair, eyelashes, and eyebrows. She had a sense of humor, which I believe can be an asset in times like these.

Karen mentioned that she had gone wig shopping, but they were a bit out of her price range and then went on to say, "I've heard that they are itchy and uncomfortable too. It was a challenge in the beginning, losing my hair that is, but I got over my ego and I feel pretty good about myself now." I loved her attitude; it was inspiring and convicting.

She was very honest with me and told me her experience was very hard, but she was a fighter and was determined to stay strong and give the battle all she had. I must admit, that as she was sharing, there were moments when I was doing all I could to not shed a tear. I was taking deep but quiet breaths and trying to blow air up towards my eyes to prevent the tears from flowing.

As I reflect back on the many visits to the hospital for both ourselves and to do pastoral visits for others, I have had to fight back many emotions triggered by all I would witness that would cause tears to flow.

Karen shared that her spouse had left her during this process, as he could not handle what she was going through, a narrative I later came to find out was more common than I would have ever imagined.

Our time had come to see the doctors. Doug's name was called and off we went. With every step we took, we were that much closer to understanding what the immediate future held for us as a family, and what course Doug would take to encounter his healing.

Regardless of the report in the natural, we knew where our hope came from. We would hold on to the Report of the Lord through it all. There are many wonderful and very gifted doctors and medical teams. Yet the Great Physician Himself is the One we trusted, leading the way.

Once we settled in the designated examination room, we met with various doctors and staff. They shared the results of the tests, and gave us more instructions. I walked out with a feeling of disbelief. *How did we not catch this sooner? Is this really happening?* And most importantly, *God, we trust You and need You.* Psalm 46:1 says, *"God is our refuge and strength."* We walked away from the office and into the hospital corridors knowing He was and would be our refuge and strength.

The late Leonard Ravenhill had written Doug a note that he has held dear to his heart. It reads, "Dearest Brother Doug, let others live on the raw or cutting edge, you and I must live on the edge of eternity." Doug is always concerned about those who don't know our Heavenly Father. He wants others to experience the life-changing freedom that comes with a relationship with the Lord.

I have heard him in deep intercession in the middle of the night crying out to the Lord for our nation and for our leaders, both in the church and in politics. He is one who teaches us to take the high road and often that comes at a cost. Doug has been a good example to our family and those who have walked close enough to observe him and he reminds us that we should live each moment uprightly and without regrets regarding our future and eternity. It is because of this that I can say this is not the end, only the beginning of a new chapter to a story that will someday be entitled, "A Life Well Lived."

We knew our friends were waiting to hear from us via social media and email. The following is what we posted after having received a clearer understanding of what was taking place in Doug's body.

Facebook post from June 4:

Today would be a bittersweet day. The day we had been waiting for finally came; we would know the extent of the diagnosis and the name and details of the battle we were thrust into. We woke up strong in the Lord and

as ready as anyone could be to face what lay ahead; however, once you step foot in MD Anderson, the reality of
the hurt many are going through hits you and it is hard
not to be moved emotionally. Our heartfelt compassion
goes out to all those who are contending for their own
breakthroughs. Our admiration goes out to the staff of
this healing center.

We have decided to look at the cup half full as
opposed to half empty. With this in mind, let me share
with you the diagnosis that many who are joining us on
this journey have been waiting for. We will start with
the positive. The cancer is not in his bone marrow, nor is
it in his brain. This was a big concern and we are beyond
thankful to the Lord for the good news. Now for the
prayer contending news: Doug has been diagnosed with
Stage 4 large B-cell lymphoma. We are needing to do
another biopsy as soon as possible to determine which
of two protocols his attending physicians will choose.
The cancer has spread to his liver, chest, abdomen, and
throughout his body. Interestingly, the blood work
shows that all the organs are working perfectly and his
t-cell counts and immune system are working well. This
is good news. We are contending with a very aggressive
cancer, but it can be fought aggressively. Our trust is in
the Lord, and we truly have a peace in the midst of this
storm.

The Bible says that the prayers of the righteous avail
much. We are confident that they have been heard, and
they will continue to be heard, as you all join us in praying for a complete healing. We are expectant of a miracle, as we know that there is nothing impossible for our
God.

We will travel as planned to The Response South Carolina where Doug will be facilitating again. We will join thousands in prayer, worship, and fastedness, and saturate heaven for our nation and nations of the world. Praise will be on our lips. Shortly after our return, they are anticipating starting Doug on chemotherapy. All is truly in God's hands. We cannot thank you all enough for your love and prayers. We are beyond blessed and without words. As you pray for us, please don't forget to pray for the many who don't have a support system or knowledge of the Lord.

May they have amazing encounters with the Living God. Through this journey, may we also let His life and light shine in and through us in such a way that others may be drawn to Him. We know that the Great Physician, Himself, is overseeing the whole process! Isaiah 26:3: *You will keep him in perfect peace, whose mind is stayed on You, because he trusts in You.* #DougBeatsCancer #StringerStrong #OurGodReigns

After making the above post, the prayers and well wishes only increased. With that came more suggestions for treatment, recommendations for supplements, special diets to help fight cancer, and an outpouring of love.

Life was busy and now we had something added to our schedule that would take precedence over most of what we had to steward. We needed time to take it all in and process what we had been told. That time came in the evenings and early mornings, as each of us would go into our prayer closets or respective areas to just be alone with God and process our feelings and racing thoughts.

In some ways, I believe that Doug's determination and drive to keep his commitments were part of his strategic plan. Not everyone will be able to do the same, for various reasons, the biggest being physical limitations due to the side effects of the cancer or the treatment.

"I'VE COME TOO FAR TO QUIT NOW"

Doug coined a phrase from an experience he had while attending high school in Japan at an American military base. He was competing in the Far East High School Wrestling Tournament and was expected to take first in his weight class. On the first day of the competition, he fractured his left elbow. His sensei (coach) wrapped his arm and had him ice it throughout the night. The next day, his sensei asked him if he wanted to continue or quit. Doug thought about it for a moment, and then replied, "Sensei, I've come too far to quit now." That very message is one that has carried him through various pitfalls and valleys in life. His desire to win had become greater than his moments of pain or challenge.

I have heard him say in pulpits all over the world, "In Christ, there are no giants too big, no challenges, obstacles, or temptations we cannot overcome. Are you willing to let God do His big job in the world through you? Can your desire to be a champion for Christ overcome the challenges and fears you face? With His empowering, we can." And there's a phrase known as a Stringerism that has lit fires under many people, young and old alike: "May your desire to win always be greater than your moments of pain and challenge." Doug ended up taking first place in Japan and second in all the Far East during the competition—all with a fractured elbow. Philippians 4:13 says, *I can do all things through Christ who strengthens me.* His desire to win was greater than his moment of challenge.

Doug had determined in his heart and mind that he would face this medical challenge as just that: a challenge. He would not be subdued by the diagnosis; instead he would quiet his spirit, hear from God and be obedient to His instruction, with His encouragement. We would hold on to our vision of hope that would keep us focused on our desired destination.

5

THROUGH THE STORM

Within forty-eight hours of the Stage 4 diagnosis, we were at MD Anderson for a full day of testing. I chose to join Doug on every appointment, whether it was for scans, tests, blood work, or chemotherapy infusions. It was important for me that Doug did not feel he was going at this alone. Yes, he had the love and support of his friends and co-laborers, but I needed him to be confident that his wife would be by his side every step of the way. I did not want him to sense any negative emotion, signs of exhaustion, fear, or weakness on my part.

Yes, I experienced all of the above, and undoubtedly, I realized I couldn't hide every feeling or challenge from him. I just didn't want him to worry about my physical and emotional health. Nothing I was going through could compare to the load Doug was carrying. I have heard it said that having emotional support minimizes the patient's psychological stress. I was intentional to communicate support for him in every way possible.

TEARS HARD TO CONTROL

The last test of the day was a biopsy of the growth on the right side of his neck—now the size of a large avocado. Doug was taken back to the surgical area; Ashley and I would wait for a few hours before being called back to see him. I spent some of this time with my laptop open, reading more about lymphoma cancer and the possible protocols that would be used to treat Doug. Ashley was focused on her homeschool assignments. Her back was to me, so she could not see the tears that began to stream down my face as my body released tension from sentiments I had been trying to contain.

The day before, Doug and I had driven outside of Houston to visit a long-time friend of the ministry who was given a few days to a few weeks to live. She had battled cancer for years and had experienced many moments of victory. Barring a miracle of the Lord, her greatest victory would come when she entered the portals of eternity and met her Savior face to face.

I was moved to tears when I saw this frail, bald, weak princess of the King pray for Doug. She could barely be heard; her voice was like a soft whisper. I was on my knees next to Doug who held her and her husband's hands as they agreed in prayer. Seeing her depleted was very hard for me, but witnessing Doug pray for her and her corresponding with him was a priceless treasure. Here were two people in a fight for their lives praying for each other; I simply could not control my tears.

Perhaps all of this, along with seeing the many taxed people around me at the hospital, is what caused the slow stream of tears to flow freely down my face in public. It was not uncommon to look around and see people misty-eyed on occasion. Some were obviously patients, others family or friends. Having spoken to some of the patients, I must say the tears were often not of sadness, but of discomfort or pain caused by the disease or the effects of their medication. It was simply a reality of life and the consequences of what each was living out, not by choice, but by circumstance.

I continued to research as much as I could in every spare moment, regularly reading up on the many recommendations that had been suggested. The information on the medications, side effects, procedures, and protocols that could possibly be used was more than my heart could bear at the time. I was having a very sentimental day and could not bring the tears under control, so I chose to reach out to two mighty women of God, both of whom were in similar battles, together with their husbands. Each of them had reached out to me, but up until this point, I had not asked many questions, as I did not know what we were facing. Both of their husbands were being treated at MD Anderson for either reoccurring cancer or follow-up protocol. They unselfishly shared their knowledge and advice, and their encouragement was a priceless treasure. Each of them will forever be heroes in my heart.

The Bible says in 1 Corinthians 10:13 that God never gives us more tests or temptations beyond what we can handle, yet at this time, I felt like I couldn't handle much more. When I took the time to look up from my computer screen, I saw patients waiting to be called back for their tests; some looked feeble, delicate, and run-down. It was a reminder of how blessed many of us are to have our health, limbs, family, and friends.

THE WORDS OF JESUS IN MATTHEW 11:28 ARE A GAME-CHANGER AND AN AWESOME REVELATION THAT CAN HELP YOU SHIFT YOUR PERSPECTIVE AND STATE OF MIND.

In the midst of it all, God was ministering to my heart and soul. Suddenly a verse given to me the night before became very real to me; it was a word in season. Jesus says in Matthew 11:28 (NIV), *"Come to me, all you who are weary and burdened, and I will give you rest."* At that moment, I figured out what God was saying to me; it was a game-changer and an awesome revelation that would shift my perspective and present state of mind.

FOCUS MOVES TO MISSION FIELD

My eyes were no longer looking at sick patients and their caregivers, but instead they were focused on a mission field. I began to declare life over every person who had the dreaded patient wristband on—and they were all around me. I declared healing on earth for each of them and revelation of the Lord should they not know Him. Joy was returning and I could breathe with ease once more. My focus was no longer on me or my circumstances, but on how I could be a blessing to others; I had peace beyond human comprehension. Go, God!

At last, Doug was settled into a private room for those coming out of surgery. Ashley and I were called back to enjoy his company until they could release him to go home. Ashley was singing praise songs and dancing around the room, full of joy for her Dad. She believed all that she was witnessing was just part of the healing process. In her mind, his healing would come; it was not an option. Ashley loves to hug us and that day, she leaned over Doug's hospital bed and held on to him tightly.

They are two of a kind, both cut from the same piece of cloth, and God used our daughter's bubbly personality and faith to change the atmosphere in the patient holding room. I walked into the hospital sad on the inside and tired on the outside, but I walked out optimistic. That was something only God could do. Psalm 30:11 (GNT) says, *"You have changed my sadness into a joyful dance; you have taken away my sorrow and surrounded me with joy."* God used Ashley's childlike faith and the joy within her to truly surround Doug and me with much-needed promise. I had an attitude of gratitude in the midst of what seemed like a dangerous storm. As we left the hospital that evening, Doug prayed, as he often had since the diagnosis, that the Big C (Christ Jesus) was bigger than the little c, cancer. He thanked God for the hospital, the team of doctors caring for him, and his healing.

We fully chose to embrace the meaning behind the hashtags that we and others began to use: "Doug Beats Cancer" and "Stringer Strong." We would pray and believe for His will and the best outcome. I would cry, wipe my tears, have moments of strength and joy, and then, when I least expected it, I would cry again. It was all part of the process.

After the biopsy results came in, it was determined which of the two protocols of chemotherapy Doug would be assigned. By the grace of God, he would not be hospitalized every few weeks for the infusion. He would receive it as an outpatient. This would essentially mean that each time he was scheduled for treatment, he would go to the hospital two days in a row. One of those two days would be an all-day affair. We were grateful because Lord allowing, Doug would be able to continue ministering and serving as his heart desired and as much as he was physically able to handle.

CHEMOTHERAPY...OR DEATH

When Doug was initially told about the chemotherapy, I recall how he looked at the doctor and boldly asked, "What would happen if I chose not to take the chemo?"—a question, I am sure, that many patients ask. Knowing all the side effects, both short- and long-term, would warrant that question from just about everyone. With a stoic face, the doctor looked him in the eyes and said, "Let me put it this way: if you choose not to take the treatment plan, you will be a patient here in a couple of months looking for emergency care."

When the doctor said Doug's cancer was 80 percent aggressive, I understood in greater measure what he meant. We were in a race against time. At this point, it was not a question for me what Doug should do as he had to make that decision himself. I am grateful that he didn't shut me out and allowed me to be a part of the decision process. He took my feelings into consideration and trusted that I was praying and hearing from God as well.

GOD'S IN CHARGE OF PRAYER GATHERING

Within a few days, our family flew to Charleston, South Carolina, for The Response Prayer gathering, where both Governors Bobby Jindal of Louisiana and Nikki Haley of South Carolina were present. We were determined to honor our commitment to continue serving by the grace of God. It was a powerful time of prayer and worship. In retrospect, we realized how impactful and providential The Response South Carolina was on many levels. We also recognized the providence of God, even through the unexpected challenges we were facing.

Doug and the team had worked to bring the churches together to pray for their state and the nation at this gathering. Putting all their differences aside and meeting at the cross of Christ, the pastors crossed racial, denominational, and generational lines as they encouraged their congregants to join us.

Originally, the event was going to be held in Columbia, which is more centrally located. Greenville was also considered. But adequate facilities were not available in either city on that day, so it was decided to hold it in Charleston, along the coast.

For six hours, more than 4,000 people took part in this solemn assembly of prayer, fasting, and worship, joined by multiple thousands more around the globe via television and livestreaming online. Relationships were forged and healing took place.

Four days later, nine people were killed in a mass shooting at Mother Emanuel AME Church in the heart of Charleston. We heard from many pastors and leaders in the community that the obedience of The Response's leadership team in carrying out the responsibility yielded what a nation witnessed. As Doug said, "Churches came out...arm in arm together, praying and singing and standing with Mother Emanuel AME Church. And what could have been a greater tragedy...turned into a message of a larger context." The message of forgiveness from the victims' families reverberated across America.

Dr. Gary Miller of the American Renewal Project told *The Washington Times*, "Hindsight provides the insight to see why God's hand guided this prayer event to Charleston four days before the tragedy. There could not have been a more strategic location for it."[1]

Doug refused to let the enemy defeat him, which enabled him to be a part of something that helped to bring hope and healing in a very difficult situation. Governor Haley's pastor told Doug, "We couldn't get through this if it wasn't for the gathering of all the churches in prayer, crossing their barriers... thousands locked arm in arm, singing and praying."

STILL DEALING WITH CANCER...

A day before the church shooting, we were scheduled to return to Houston. We had an early Monday morning

---

1. W. Scott Lamb, "The tie that binds: Charleston and prayer in the aftermath," *The Washington Times*, June 24, 2015 (www.washingtontimes.com/news/2015/jun/24/tie-binds-charleston-and-prayer-aftermath-tragedy).

appointment at the hospital so Doug could start chemother-apy. Doug would have a PICC line placed in the bicep area of his right arm. PICC is an acronym for percutaneously inserted central catheter, a medical device that is placed into a vein to allow access to the bloodstream. Pronounced "pick," it allows fluids and medications to be given to a patient. This would be a permanent fixture until the end of Doug's treatment, allowing the medical team to infuse the chemo and anything else needed.

Once at the airport, we encountered flight delays because of both mechanical issues and bad weather. Finally, our plane departed for Washington, D.C., where we would make our con-nection to Houston. Once we landed, we were told there was a mechanical delay with the connecting aircraft. We were con-cerned as weather reports showed severe weather in Houston and the potential of a tropical storm. After hours upon hours at the airport, we were told our flight was canceled. *This could not be happening!* We needed to get back to Houston. Time was of the essence to get the PICC line in and the treatment started.

We were able to book a room at a nearby hotel. We checked in after 1:30 a.m. and would only be in the room for about three hours before catching the shuttle bus back to the airport to board the first flight departing for Houston. We contemplated sleeping at the airport, but decided that a few hours in a bed, along with a shower, would be the best choice.

Once we landed, we did not have enough time to go home, so we ate some breakfast and headed for the hospital. The streets were somewhat desolate as people were preparing for the storm and many were advised not to leave their homes unless absolutely necessary. Our being at the hospital for the PICC line placement was absolutely necessary.

Ashley and I sat down while Doug checked himself in. After a short while, he was called back and we asked if we could join him. In fact, the nurse allowed us to watch a video with him that was required to be seen prior to the procedure that would take place. This video included information about the potential risks.

BUT WHAT ABOUT THE RISK?

I know the hospital has to do their due diligence and warn us of possible outcomes, but oh my goodness, talk about the emotional impact it had on me. I was sitting on the gurney behind Doug, when tears began to flow. I wiped them as quickly as I could and tried to be as still as I could so that neither he nor Ashley would notice. After a quick, "So long," as I could hardly look Doug in the face for fear of the floodgates opening, I rushed out of the room, leaving Doug alone with the medical staff.

I recall so vividly how I had a total meltdown in the garden area on an upper level of the hospital. Initially, Ashley and I sat in the waiting area, but the video and the risks mentioned kept playing in my head. I could not hold back the tears. Ashley asked me what was wrong and for a long while, I could not even get words out since I have occasional struggles with asthma and I could feel an attack coming on.

The emotional reaction to the video was triggering a physical reaction of stress and I had to leave. I walked toward the outdoor garden and found a seat where people couldn't see me crying. Ashley followed me out and tried to comfort me. In some ways, it breaks my heart that I put her through that; it was as though our roles were reversed. She was the one speaking life over me, praying and doing everything she could to console me. The winds outside were grating and blowing cool air. I needed to control myself, but was not finding success fast enough.

I pulled out my cell phone and called my mother. I always try to be strong for mom and can only recall one other time I cried like that in front of her. I recall her answering the phone while I struggled to speak, as I was sobbing uncontrollably.

With a very concerned voice, she replied, "What happened? Is Doug okay?"

"Yes," I responded.

"Are you all okay?"

"Yes." I had great difficulty getting the words out as I told her about the video we had just seen and the concern and fear that had suddenly set in. I asked her a few questions about my dad and his journey with pancreatic cancer. That morning, we connected in a way I would have never imagined. I realized I could relate to her not just as my mother, or as a fellow mother and wife. Now we could relate in a new, unexpected, and unwelcome way: cancer had invaded the bodies of both our spouses.

DAD STOPPED HIS CHEMO

My dad was a warrior, a strong, determined, and able man, but after having chemo treatment, he chose to suspend the protocol. Dad said the side effects were more than he could or wanted to handle. His short-lived journey with cancer was a very difficult one and the only cancer experience my mom had ever had until now. She agreed with me in prayer that Doug's experience would be different as would be the outcome. We prayed together, pouring our hearts out to God, and with the strong winds that occasionally whistled through the garden, the fears were blown away.

I began once again to take control of my heart and mind. The outcome was silence in His embrace. All along, Ashley sat quietly in intercession for me, occasionally rubbing my back, giving me hugs, and just loving me through the juncture I found myself in.

By the grace of God, mom's and Ashley's love and prayers, and a few cold-water face washes in the ladies' restroom, the evidence of my broken and concerned heart was concealed. The only thing I wanted Doug to notice was a wife ready to go home and enjoy his company, along with a nap, before the start of chemo the following day.

When Doug eventually stepped out into the waiting room, he did so with gauze wrapped around the PICC line that was now a temporary fixture in his body until the treatment was completed. Everything was becoming more real and tangible.

With the storm on the horizon, after unloading our suitcases, our first mission was to secure anything outside that could fly off and do damage to our home or a neighbor's. Immediately afterward, Doug called the family together for a time of prayer and communion.

A TIME TO BE GRATEFUL

He reminded us of the importance of spiritual preparation, saying it is often only fully realized or recognized through crisis and challenging situations. We had much to be thankful for and he wanted to make sure that before we all became occupied with our to-do list, we could have an intimate time with the Lord as a family. He asked each of us to name at least three things we were grateful for. Perspectives change when you look at things through the lens of gratitude. We have to be intentional to always recognize that life is a gift and each day is a privilege to experience.

> PERSPECTIVES CHANGE WHEN YOU LOOK AT THINGS THROUGH THE LENS OF GRATITUDE. WE HAVE TO BE INTENTIONAL TO RECOGNIZE THAT LIFE IS A GIFT AND EACH DAY IS A PRIVILEGE TO EXPERIENCE.

Doug began by saying, "I am grateful that one of the titles that God gives Himself is, '*Father of mercies and God of all comfort,*' who comforts us in all our tribulations, troubles, and trials (2 Corinthians 1:3–4). No matter what we are going through, we must remember this attribute of God's character in our lives, and also remember what Paul reminds us of in 2 Corinthians 2:14—God *always* leads us into triumph through Christ Jesus."

He set the tone for us to have an attitude of gratitude. We talked about the many blessings we had—a roof over our head, protection from the imminent storm, we made it back in time for treatment to begin, being at our hospital of choice with a great medical team to oversee the protocol, praying friends, food in the pantry, cars in the garage, and having each other. Most of all, we had Hope; His name was and is Jesus.

Up until now, I had not shared an additional circumstance that was tugging at my heart and playing a role on my seesaw of emotions. Ashley had been diagnosed with a variety of physical challenges throughout her young life. She has had to deal with many food allergies, irritable bowel syndrome (IBS), and other distracting diagnoses. The only day available for her to have an exploratory procedure that would require complete sedation was on the day that Doug would start his chemo. My heart was torn as I wanted to be there for both of them; in addition, Doug wanted to be present for Ashley as well. In the end, moving either of their procedures would not be an option.

FRIEND STEPS IN TO HELP

I thank God for the body of Christ that was there for us in our time of need. A friend and co-laborer, Rick Torrison, volunteered to pick up Doug at our home at 6:15 a.m. and take him to the hospital for a full day of chemo and more. Ashley and I departed our home at 5:30 a.m. to check into Texas Children's

Hospital in the Medical Center, just a few buildings over from where Doug would be.

After settling into the hospital room and in between the many nurses and medical staff who would come and check on Ashley, ask questions, and do pre-op procedures, I sensed a need to distract her from all that was going on in her midst. Thus, I tried engaging her on various topics, but with the reality of what she and her father were going through, I don't know that I did a very good job because she asked me to please be quiet. I laugh now, but I wasn't laughing then.

The hospital staff was fantastic and it was obvious they were used to dealing with children who were scared or in pain. The anesthesiologist came to put the IV in for Ashley and began to apply some medication to relax her and numb the area where the IV would be put in.

It is most unfortunate, but she has been told she has rolling veins. In thirteen years of life, she had not experienced one nurse or physician who was able to draw blood on the first try. In fact, it usually took five or more attempts and a few times, an ultrasound machine was needed to find a potential vein. Needless to say, I could never tell her if we were scheduled to have her blood drawn, or she would not have willingly gone into the doctor's office, at least not without my having to be stern with her.

This time was no different; they were not finding success and this was making her uncomfortable. Tears began to stream, which eventually became a full cry, "Mommy, please help me. Make them stop." She had desired to take a Somebody Cares Bear with her as it was her way of having Doug near. She was squeezing the bear tightly and asking me to take her to her father.

The medical staff asked if they could program the television in her room to cartoons or a movie to distract her, but she said,

"No, I want to hear worship music." I pulled out my cell phone, played her requested song, and God ministered to her, me, and the staff. After the team left, one of the nurses came back in and told her, "I am a Christian, too. You have nothing to worry about; you will be okay." I thanked him and Ashley began to talk to him about Jesus. In retrospect, I believe she was internalizing her concerns or fears over all that was going on in her life and perhaps that played a part in her being less tolerant of the pain or inconvenience.

ANOTHER FRIEND SHOWS UP

After numerous unsuccessful attempts to get the IV in, the anesthesiologist offered me another solution. I would go down with her to the operating room and be there with her while they put the mask on her face and the sedation took effect. Susie Wolf, one of my dearest friends and sisters in the Lord, who is also a chaplain, showed up at the hospital. Her timing was perfect. We walked alongside Ashley's gurney and some of the medical team. When the automatic doors opened up to what felt like a very big operating room, my heart was overwhelmed. I had been holding Ashley's hand the entire time. There had to be ten people inside. There was a wall with windows and people wearing scrubs on the other side with computers and medical equipment all around. Houston has many teaching hospitals and I believe I was told that was the reason for the extra people in the rooms.

It was obvious that Ashley was uneasy while lying there, surrounded by strangers wearing surgical masks and bright lights shining down on her. Her doctor approached her and asked a few questions. She shared that she was a singer/songwriter and had written a few songs and asked the team if she could sing a song for them. The doctor graciously agreed. And so, lying on a gurney as people moved about and prepared for her procedure, Ashley began to sing a verse. Peace had settled in her heart. The team affirmed her. With that, the anesthesiologist explained that he would be putting a mask on her and she was to take a few deep breaths.

Within a few moments, she released my hand as she was successfully sedated. Fighting back the tears, I walked away, trusting that the Physician of all physicians was in the room with her, overseeing the process. My friend Susie chose to remain with me the entire time.

We spent some of the time in the hospital chapel, where we interceded for both Doug and Ashley's healing. This would mark another moment in time where I was emotionally spent and recognized that the only way to overcome my grief was by dependence on God, my Strong Tower.

Psalm 107:19–21 says:

Then they cried out to the Lord in their trouble, and He saved them out of their distresses. He sent His word and healed them, and delivered them from their destructions. Oh, that men would give thanks to the Lord for His goodness.

God used Susie to infuse me with His much-needed love that morning in a way that I didn't realize I would need. She prayed with me, listened to me, and regularly reminded me that God was in control. Too often, many of us shut out friends or family because we don't want to become a burden to them. As I reflect on that day and many after that, I am ever grateful that we never had to experience any of the process alone. We always had friends and spiritual family to stand or sit with us. I will forever remember the kind gestures and I will forever pay it forward for as long as I have life and health.

After a lengthy time in the recovery room, Ashley was released from the hospital. It was just past midday and the only thing she wanted to do was go see Daddy. She was still quite groggy when we arrived at MD Anderson, so we were offered a wheelchair for her to get around. As it turned out, Doug had yet to have his treatment started. He was awaiting the meeting with the attending doctor prior to beginning.

LAUGHING, JOKING...AND WAITING

Susie was kind enough to sit with Ashley as I made my way back to the patient's room, where Doug and our friends were. Everyone was in good spirits; there was some laughing, joking, and words of love sprinkled in between. Everyone wanted to know how Ashley was doing, but I wanted to know about Doug first. Our attending physician was in Switzerland for a conference and the doctor assigned to Doug that day was Japanese. Doug loved it because he could talk about food and other commonalities. In fact, he told the doctor that I wouldn't eat natto with him. The doctor got a chuckle out of that and told me I was missing out. For those of you who are unfamiliar with this traditional Japanese food, natto is fermented soybeans and is known for its sticky texture and pungent smell. I have been told it is an acquired taste...and I am not willing to acquire it. Dr. Yasuhiro Oki eventually shared the must-knows and went over last-minute details before releasing Doug to be infused with the chemotherapy, which would take place in an adjacent building.

We were reminded of the risks of the protocol he would be receiving. I was pulled aside this morning as well and was told the same with Ashley before they began. The hospital staff is required to share all the side effects and worst-case scenarios. I have to admit, though, I didn't want to hear any more about what could go wrong. This time, however, I felt empowered by

His love. I had just witnessed God care for Ashley in her time of need. Now in Doug's time of need, I had peace and a renewed trust in the Lord.

Perhaps my time of rawness and prayer in the chapel earlier with Susie was a game-changer. Susie gave me a Scripture that day, Matthew 6:34 (NIV): *"Therefore do not worry about tomorrow, for tomorrow will worry about itself. Each day has enough trouble of its own."* With that in mind, I was not going to worry about what *could* happen. I would trust God had it under control and as for today, we needed to move forward, marching onward with faith that moved mountains and peace that surpassed understanding. (See Matthew 17:20; Philippians 4:7.)

Before the end of the meeting, I remember Doug telling the doctor that maybe we should just move the chemo to another day. You see, he had checked into the hospital by 7 a.m. It was now after midday. I think Doug was looking for any way out of receiving the chemo, which I totally understand. I will never forget Dr. Oki's response. He said, "If you don't start treatment now, you will be an emergency case in a very short time. Your organs will have begun to shut down, and you will have lost your appetite and lots of weight." I didn't let the doctor finish; I interrupted him and said, "He will begin today!" I wanted my husband to live and according to the doctor, we didn't have time to spare.

6

OUR LIFE MESSAGE GROWS

In the previous twenty-four hours, we had taken a flight from Washington, D.C., to Houston, had the PICC line placement, prepared for a storm, Ashley had an exploratory procedure done, and Doug was preparing for his first chemotherapy treatment—all of this with limited sleep or rest. It makes me tired just recalling the journey of that twenty-four-hour window.

That day, we were asked to make a decision regarding a necessary protocol regarding the maintenance of the PICC line. We were given an option to either come to the hospital to have the PICC line flushed daily or a caregiver of his choice could take a class on how to flush the lines as well as change the dressing, which had to be cleaned and replaced on a weekly basis, unless a sooner change was warranted. Taking into consideration the distance to the hospital from our home, the parking expense that would add up, and our time spent to and from the hospital, the answer was clear: I would take the class and be the primary person assigned to care for Doug's PICC line.

A CLASS ON THE PICC LINE

I was told that the prescription for the dressing changes and flushing solution would not be released to me until I completed a two-day class with detailed instructions on the "how to." There was a class available that afternoon. Ashley needed to be with me, so she and I left Doug with our friends and headed for the wing of the hospital where the class was taught. I wheeled her in and chose a seat in the very back.

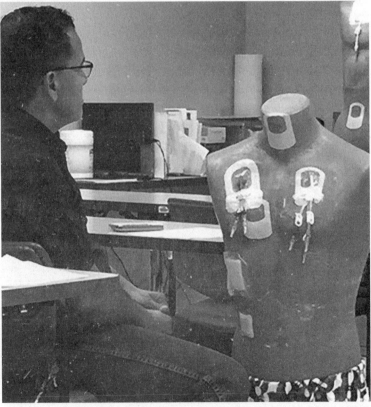

The Stringers' friend and ministry co-worker Ruben Sanchez took the class on PICC line protocols so he could serve as a backup for Lisa.

Feeling physically tired and not knowing what to expect, I wanted to be as invisible as possible. Ashley insisted on being a part of the class, so I removed the chair next to me and put her wheelchair in its place. I was blessed beyond measure when I saw a dear friend walk into the classroom. Ruben Sanchez has been a part of the ministry that we steward for over thirty years and is also Doug's spiritual son and dear friend. He showed up at the hospital early that morning to be with Doug as treatment began. We were unaware of all the pre-chemo appointments and because of them, the infusion had not yet begun so Ruben chose to join us in taking the class. He would make himself available should I be unable to do the required protocol for Doug on any given day.

I remember looking at each person as they entered the classroom and took their seats, wondering what their stories were. I would soon find out, as some of them shared about their loved ones. They came from all over the world and represented all age groups. Everyone present had someone they loved or desired to help through their battle with cancer. We were all at the beginning of the journey, or newly assigned to help in the midst of their loved one's treatment. Concern was evident on everyone's face; some looked lost, others tired, and the look of heavy hearts overshadowed any possible joy at that moment.

The class consisted of video lessons, in-class instruction, and hands-on training with dummies. As one of the first videos played, I looked over at Ashley, whose head was slumped over in her chair, sound asleep. God bless her, she was out like a light, and rightfully so. The anesthesia from earlier that morning was likely still causing her fatigue. Truth be told, I was fighting back the heavy eyelids myself. When the lights came on after the first video, Ashley apologized and asked why I let her sleep. I signaled to her to please be quiet as I needed to pay attention to every detail of the training. Somehow, she managed to stay awake for the remaining of the videos and teaching, as she was determined to learn and help in any way possible.

Because a PICC line has a high infection risk, a lot of emphasis is placed on the proper way to wash your hands and prevent the spread of germs. We were reminded that the care must be executed properly and were instructed on how to flush the PICC line with a heparin or saline solution. We also learned how to change the catheter's injection caps and the dressing. This was a lot to take in. If I were not as emotionally attached to the patient and a bit on the tired side, I think the class would have been easy to handle. It was overly stressed that we must be ever so careful to keep everything sterile. Preventing infection was the key.

SAFEGUARDING THE IMMUNE SYSTEM

Most chemotherapy patients have a compromised immune system. Their ability to fight off disease or sickness is not easy and not always successful. The teaching team notably and regularly emphasized the importance of not contributing to the introduction of germs that could cause infection to the patient. Those with a PICC line cannot swim or soak in a tub as it is very important to keep the entry area dry. Taking baths or showers required all of the connections to be completely covered, usually with a plastic wrap. This would become a burdensome chore in and of itself.

One of the points highly stressed was regarding the use of the sterile gloves. We were given step by step instructions on how to complete the assignment. There is a point when one opens a dressing change package that contains sterile gloves. You are told to put them on before touching any of the other materials in the package. The inside of the cuff of one glove is turned up, so this allows you to grab it with one hand and put it on, never touching the outside of the glove with your bare hands; thus, the materials in the kit remain sterile. It is stressed not to touch the outside of the package or anything other than the contents of the package once the gloves are on your hands. I think I have given you an idea of the magnitude of importance emphasized to the caregivers regarding learning proper protocol for dressing changes and the flushing of the line or lines.

Once the three of us completed the class, we joined Doug and Rick as it was time to start the infusion. Doug was assigned to a private room and off we went. It was obvious he was not thrilled about what was close at hand, yet that didn't mean Doug was without faith or lacking a positive attitude. He never complained or expressed fear. The only words out of his mouth were declarations of life, peace, and his trust in the Lord. I recall him walking down the long hallway to his assigned room with his lips tightly together, giving me a partial smile. Doug usually walks fast, but this time, the regular pep wasn't in his step. We all tried to keep the atmosphere light and jovial, including him. First Thessalonians 5:16–19 says, *"Rejoice always, pray without ceasing, in everything give thanks; for this is the will of God in Christ Jesus for you. Do not quench the Spirit."*

We tried to do just that. Once settled in the room, the nurse warned Doug that he would begin the infusion slowly as many people have a reaction to it within the first fifteen minutes. He scanned Doug's identification bracelet and went to get the fluids that would go into his PICC line. Prior to beginning the infusion, we took communion and prayed that nothing would enter in his body without first being washed by the blood of Jesus. Our prayer times were always powerful, comforting, strengthening, and game-changing. We prayed from the depths of our hearts and always quoted Scripture. That day, it was Psalm 121:1–2:

"I will lift up my eyes to the hills—from whence comes my help? My help comes from the LORD, who made heaven and earth."

R-CHOP SIDE EFFECTS

The infusion began. I recall watching ever so closely as the medication began to drip from the bag with a steady flow and make its way down the line and into Doug's body. The chemo he was assigned had a few nicknames; some referred to it as R-CHOP and others called it red devil. R-CHOP is an acronym for the drugs used, while the other name refers to its deep red color and potentially dangerous side effects.

I recall the tears that flowed down my cheeks as I read about the chemotherapy and the side effects, which included hair loss, short-term memory loss, nausea, loss of appetite, bone and muscle pain, loss of sleep, sweats, mouth sores, loss of the sense of taste, and a heightened sense of smell, to name a few. Curiosity got the best of me, as I recall looking at photos of people who had been given the chemotherapy treatment. Needless to say, I was hurting for them and hurting at the possibility that my husband would experience any of the same reactions.

I sat on the edge of the hospital bed and watched with Doug as the R-CHOP entered his body. I recall holding his hand and praying as it entered in. We all declared the healing blood of Jesus is what would flow through his body and nothing else. After a short while, I decided to take Ashley with me to the waiting area, giving Doug some time with his friends.

Shortly afterward, Rick came out and offered to take Ashley home, as we were told Doug would likely be there until at least 10 p.m. She tried to convince us that we should let her stay, but her tired eyes needed rest. Considering the long and full day she had already experienced, we sent her home.

I remained in the waiting area, where very few people remained. As it was, the bad weather kept even hospital staff away that day. I had begun to write a post to update the many who had sent me messages inquiring about Doug and Ashley, when I looked up and saw a dear friend and pediatric oncologist at MD Anderson, Dr. Dean Lee. He took the time to come see us before heading home for the day. I walked him back to Doug's room, where Ruben excused himself to get coffee and give us time alone with Dean. I'll never forget the unexpected conversation. Simply put, he was real with us. He was better than Google, as he shared his heart and brought up things I hadn't yet thought about or had a good understanding of. I recall his glossy eyes as he prayed for us and bid us a good night.

Ruben would return to the room with his wife, Cynthia, and would remain with us until the infusion was complete and we were sent home, which was nearly midnight.

I eventually posted the update on social media and closed with this paragraph:

> Like in posts past, Doug and I recognize that there are many more who are suffering greater challenges. A friend of ours just lost her young adult son a week ago. All around us are people who are weak, sick, and in need. Injustice for many is taking place all over the world, but God is more than able.

The streets were quiet and our ride home was relatively the same. We had worship music on and began to thank the Lord for all He had done for us, including the fact that we were able to go home. As we neared our home, it was obvious that Doug was not doing well. He had his head tilted back, eyes closed, and mentioned feeling a bit nauseous. He also tried to keep things light and said something that made me laugh and caused him to give me a partial smile.

NO JOKE—DOUG IS FREEZING

We pulled into the garage were greeted by Mom and Ashley as we entered the house. Ashley gave Daddy a hug, and Mom just said, "Thank you, Jesus, it is over, and you all are home safe." Doug took a seat on the couch and within moments, he said he was cold. Doug is rarely cold. I sincerely thought he was joking, as he is a practical jokester and would do or say things to change the atmosphere and distract us from worrying. We wanted to close the night out with the family gathered to say a quick prayer of thanksgiving when Doug said again, "I am not just cold, I'm freezing." I put a blanket over him, but his body was shivering uncontrollably and would not cease.

Within moments, prayer time was over and I led my blanket-wrapped husband into the bedroom. I pulled the bedding back, helped him get in bed, and tucked him in, but the intense shivering would not stop. He suggested a hot shower. I turned the hot water on and began to get the plastic wrap and other materials needed to wrap his PICC line and prevent it from getting wet. I was moving as fast as I could as his entire body was shaking profusely and to say it scared me a little is an understatement.

No matter how much I had read, nothing prepared me for what I was witnessing. It was almost as though Doug had lost control of his own body. We got through the shower, which included taking the plastic wrap off of Doug's arm very carefully, and had him tucked back in bed.

I could not put enough blankets on him to get his body to stabilize. I ran to get a trash can and put it next to the bed should the nausea overtake him and he not be able to make it to the bathroom. An hour would go by before I could put everything in order and have what I thought we needed to get us through the night. I could not imagine the night being any more difficult than it already was. Mom had not gone to bed; she was waiting for me to come out and let her know how he was doing. She had been sitting on the couch praying the entire time. I'm sure she was recalling difficult memories of her walk with Dad's cancer journey.

INFECTION CONTROL VITAL

Many articles and posts I read all mentioned the importance of keeping the patient away from anything that could make him sick. Infection control was the main goal as we were constantly warned that his suppressed immune system needed to be protected and I was determined to do that. This meant that either when he woke up or before then, I would need to go into the shower, clean it, and make it ready for him to use.

You may think, *How dirty could it have been? He doesn't work with oil or dirt.* But bacteria grows just about everywhere all the time, hence the need to take every precaution to make his environment as aseptic as possible. I put on my gloves and with my organic cleaning sprays and towels in hand, I began to scrub the tub and shower. It was the middle of the night and my day was not yet over. I was tired, and within a few hours, I would have been awake for twenty-four hours. I kept in mind that it was ever so important that I took all the precautions to keep myself healthy, too, which included getting adequate rest. If I were to get sick anytime during his treatment, it could mean that I wouldn't be able to be around him.

As I cleaned, I repeated Psalm 27:13 (NIV): *"I remain confident of this: I will see the goodness of the LORD in the land of the living.*" I scrubbed everything thoroughly, occasionally wiping my tears on my shoulders, and I repeated the verse until all was clean. I eventually crawled into bed as quietly and softly as possible as I did not want to wake him. As I laid myself to rest, I just stared at my beloved husband, repeating the psalm again and again until I fell asleep.

A NEW DIET REGIMEN

Morning came and with that came the protocol of my non-negotiable diet regimen. With all the research I had done, one of the topics we embraced was eating to live. I had mentioned previously that we were inundated with suggestions of every type to help us beat the cancer or curtail its growth with either diet plans or supplements. I narrowed our list to a manageable few. Over time, I have shared this list with people who have asked what we did in addition to the hospital's protocol. As I have said before, everyone's story, outcome, and tolerance is different, so what we did may not be conducive to all for various reasons. Nonetheless, I want to share our two lists with you.

The first is the list of items we incorporated into our diets, most certainly Doug's. The second is the food items we chose to do without. I say this with a smile on my face, as I was the one to really make the choices. Being in charge of the kitchen, I chose not to include anything that could work against all that was being done to produce healing.

If Doug had his way, he might have had snuck in some bacon a time or two. Who knows? Perhaps he did. I believe without a doubt that the diet change made a difference. Eating balanced and nutritious food can help to keep you energized. To my amazement during our journey, Doug had relatively good energy levels much of the time, and that is a big part of the battle. When you are weak and unable to do things, you give in to sleeping and are not able to produce much. Some think they are worthless during this season. Don't believe that lie.

Our heavenly Father is filled with love for you and, needless to say, I am sure there are family and friends who are hurting because *you* are hurting and are praying you through the process. John 3:16 says, *"For God so loved the world that He gave His only begotten Son, that whoever believes in Him should not perish but have everlasting life."* You are worth everything to the Creator of the universe, and your life is of great value and worth for Him, even as you are going through your moment of challenge.

> YOU ARE WORTH EVERYTHING TO THE CREATOR OF THE UNIVERSE, EVEN AS YOU ARE GOING THROUGH YOUR MOMENT OF CHALLENGE.

Regarding the diet, I have heard people on both sides of the fence, some stating diet has nothing to do with the healing of one's body, and others adamant that the diet was everything. Should you be in a cancer journey or caring for someone who is, pray about what you should do and don't share your protocol with the world. There will always be those who disagree with you. You will know who you can talk to and trust to give you good counsel. The last thing you need is added stress from others' opinions.

A NATURAL DIET FOR CANCER PATIENTS

- I had a juicer and made my own fresh-squeezed juice combinations. I also made smoothies using a blender so that I could keep all of the pulp, which is often rich in fiber. Doug drank these every day we were not on the road. I used different combinations of fruits and vegetables, such as broccoli, kale, spinach, pineapple, beets, celery, carrots, apples, and blueberries. I also included a dash of cinnamon, a dab of turmeric, and some flax seed.

+ I brewed soursop tea for Doug to start his day instead of coffee. He would have one cup in the morning and most evenings, he would have one cup before bed. Soursop is known by some practitioners of herbal medicine to treat various ailments. The fruit's anti-cancer properties have attracted much attention. It is also known as graviola tree leaves.

+ He took supplements, including a high-grade turmeric supplement daily and vitamin supplements modified to the dose the oncologist recommended.

+ Doug also drank mineral water. Initially, I made him a cup of water with a spoonful of baking soda and mixed it well, expecting him to drink it. Baking soda has an alkalizing effect and reduces acidity. Eventually, we discovered a natural mineral water product called Crazy Water that did the same thing. It comes in a few different levels; the higher the level, the worse the taste and the more effective it is.

+ Kombucha and probiotic drinks were part of his diet at least four or five times a week to help improve his immune system.

+ He drank a few tablespoons of apple cider vinegar with water on a daily basis.

FOODS TO AVOID

+ Cut out as much fatty foods as possible. If it was fried, we were likely to avoid it. We limited red meat intake and eliminated processed meats altogether, including turkey bacon.

+ We avoided excessive intake of salt and oily foods. Transfats and saturated fats were avoided as much as possible.

+ Eliminated all sugar unless it was naturally in fruit. We were intentional about not eating fruit that was high in sugar, such as figs, bananas, grapes, and mangos.

+ We avoided anything acidic, such as coffee.

SOME GOOD THINGS DON'T TASTE GOOD

Doug reminds me on occasion that when he was first diagnosed with cancer, I made a few promises that I did not keep. As I began the research on how to help beat the disease with clean eating, I presented him some of the changes I proposed making and protocols I would be implementing. Let's face it, not all the things that are good for you taste good. Sometimes, it is simply an acquired taste.

I remember ordering the soursop tea and making a cup for myself, along with Doug's, so we could enjoy it together. That lasted for less than a week. The tea is really not bad at all; I just never acquired a taste for it. Then there were the vegetable smoothies for breakfast. I excused myself from enjoying them on days that I totally missed the mark on great taste or even decent taste, sometimes using the excuse that I ran out of the ingredients, all of which could be true. I just intentionally did not make another round if I didn't like the mix of the day.

The one that takes the cake in his book is the baking soda and water mix. I told him everything he would eat and drink, we would do together. I would be right there with him every step of the way. That lasted one taste. With all sincerity, I just couldn't do it, I started gagging after just one sip. I can hear his voice in my head saying, "Honey, you promised. You said whatever I drank, you would drink. You also said we would do this together, and you are committed to what you confess."

I apologized profusely and told him that was not going to happen. He threatened me by saying, "If you don't do it, I won't do it." But he was just trying to get me to drink the crazy concoctions. In the end, Doug did everything I suggested and never objected. His only complaint was that I didn't keep my promise. He still jokes about it to this day and says I should have said, "Do as I say, not as I do."

In all seriousness, I have great admiration for him and all patients who have no choice but to submit to protocols of all types just to survive or get well. My heart goes out to the young patients and their parents or family members, many of whom, I'm sure, would gladly take protocols on behalf of their loved ones to protect them from all they endure physically and emotionally.

We were still relatively inexperienced, on a journey whose length we did not know. We wanted to believe with the many who were praying that it would be quick, but no matter the length, we were confident of this, that God was with us and that this too shall pass. We chose to encourage others as they reassured us through our journey in the valley. We also knew that through it all, we must never forget to thank God for mountaintop experiences in the past and the one in the future that we were believing for.

Joshua 1:9 (NASB) says, *"Have I not commanded you? Be strong and courageous! Do not tremble or be dismayed, for the LORD your God is with you wherever you go."* And Jeremiah 17:7 (NIV) says, *"Blessed is the one who trusts in the LORD."*

WE MUST TRUST THE LORD AT ALL TIMES

Being strong, courageous, and trusting in the Lord is always easier when things are good. But when they are bad, we must trust the same, standing strong in God's strength. Thus far, in the process of writing this book, I have recalled many tears shed throughout the journey to date. I wish I could tell you that I rarely cried, but that would be far from the truth. I had moments throughout where something would trigger a runaway tear, other times a light cry, and a few times an uncontrollable, seemingly never-ending flood. The tears are all a part of my story, a testimony of love, pain, trust, and even joy in the midst of our encountered storm. My trust in God never wavered; in fact, it was because I trusted in Him, no matter the outcome, that I was able to bounce back from the sentimental detours.

> BEING STRONG, COURAGEOUS, AND TRUSTING IN THE LORD IS ALWAYS EASIER WHEN THINGS ARE GOOD. BUT WHEN THEY ARE BAD, WE MUST TRUST THE SAME.

Doug often shares with Ashley and me that "our personal crucibles of experience can often become a tutor along our life's journey." And that "each life experience can become a life lesson that becomes a part of our life message."

This journey certainly gave us experiences, sometimes on a daily basis, that would mature us in unique ways. Until the day our time on earth is over and we enter the portals of eternity, I am sure that much of what we lived will forever be a part of our life message. God is able!

7

BETTER GOOD DAYS

Doug had the desire to get back in the gym as it is a place to release stress, and as he says, "clear his mind." He has always been one to work out a minimum of three or four times a week. Doug enjoys lifting weights and includes cardio when time permits, generally working out alone. During these workouts, he has shared that he is processing thoughts, assignments, and concerns—releasing his energy and maybe even frustration in a healthy way, and in the process, gaining from it as well. He has received many a revelation at the gym, and of course, has found plenty of opportunities to share his faith and pray for people. This season would be no different.

His physicians had recommended that he keep as much a normal a routine as his body permitted, including trips to the gym. In fact, it was suggested that he stay active so that arthritis and other joint issues would not set in because of the chemotherapy. I often think about the many opportunities he had to use the cancer as an excuse to not answer calls, emails, attend meetings, minister, take care of his family, or work out at the gym. Not Douglas! He was determined not to let cancer get the best of him. I witnessed him serving in every capacity possible, praying with those in need, offering counsel when it was sought out, and sharing His love with anyone who would listen.

It had been over three weeks since the PICC line was in, and with all that had been taking place, aside from a very hectic schedule, time had yet to permit him to enjoy a visit to the gym. In spite of all that, he was determined to make a comeback, and I would be there to witness it.

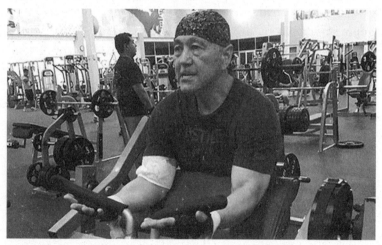

The PICC line did not stop Doug from working out.

ALL SMILES BEFORE WORKOUT

I had made some T-shirts to raise funds for the ministry that had a very popular Doug Stringer quote on them. That afternoon, he had one of the T-shirts on. He confidently walked over to me before we left the house and said, as he pointed to his chest and began to recite the quote, "See honey, my desire to win is greater than my moment of challenge!" He had the biggest smile on his face. The PICC line was nicely wrapped and protected from potential sweat that would come during the workout. He then proceeded to point out the baseball cap he had chosen to wear; it simply said, "Strength." He was ready to go.

Once at the gym, Doug was filled with joy as he was able to lift about 80 percent of his normal weights. We were able to appreciate and celebrate the smallest of successes, perhaps with a new, deeper understanding of the value of each milestone along the way. I was concerned that Doug would drive himself too hard and cause a problem with the PICC line or something else. As I expressed my concern, he looked at me and said, "Honey, today is a good day!" I knew what he was trying to tell me, so I simply smiled, shook my head, and let it go. I had to trust that Doug knew his limits and wouldn't charge beyond them. I also needed to remember and trust that God would take care of him.

Perhaps for Doug, working out was a matter of recognizing that he still had significant physical strength and ability. After all, who doesn't desire to feel accomplished or undefeated by an enemy attack? I was proud of him as he demonstrated determination. Through his actions, he motivated me in the process and reminded me not take the easy road. In fact, Doug inspired me and others not to let the little hiccups in life keep us down.

I recall noticing a very fit, middle-aged man constantly watching us during our workout. The gentleman began to approach us as Doug was doing leg extensions. I was standing next to him, cheering him on, and waiting to do my set. As he neared, he reached out, wanting to shake Doug's hand. I noticed his eyes were glossy and his voice almost cracked as he said, "Keep going! I know what you're going through and admire your perseverance. Don't quit!" Doug thanked him and we shared a few more minutes of conversation before our new friend went on his way.

At that moment, I was reminded what Doug often says, "My life is not my own." He says, "As believers in Jesus Christ, we are to reflect His love and character everywhere we go." The truth is, most of us miss the mark on a regular basis. But with intentionality, we can be a tangible expression of His love and character.

> WITH INTENTIONALITY, WE CAN BE A TANGIBLE EXPRESSION OF CHRIST'S LOVE AND CHARACTER.

In addition, Doug is a public figure and although he may not be a celebrity, he is often recognized in our city. Whether at the gym, coffeehouse, restaurant, or grocery store, not a week goes by that I don't witness a few people asking him if he is Doug Stringer. And each time, I am reminded of the responsibility we have to represent God and represent Him well.

Ephesians 5:1–2 says, *"Therefore be imitators of God as dear children. And walk in love, as Christ also has loved us and given Himself for us, an offering and a sacrifice to God for a sweet-smelling aroma."*

That day, as I looked around the gym, I could not help but think what story each person next to me had. *Do they have a spiritual or physical need? Are they walking through an emotionally difficult time?* We live in a world where we mask so much of our pain and are very quick to judge without knowing all the facts.

I pondered the importance of those of us who call upon the name of the Lord, exhibiting the fruits of the Spirit: love, joy, peace, patience, kindness, goodness, and faithfulness. I recall praying that those of us who know God would never forget that *"the name of the* LORD *is a strong tower; the righteous run to it and are safe"* (Proverbs 18:10).

CLIMBING A NEW MOUNTAIN

Doug did not have the time, energy, or physical stamina to keep up his normal workout schedule; more often than not, his spirit was willing, but he had to convince his body to agree. On another occasion, Doug, exhibiting his usual sense of humor, said he was hoping to climb a mountain. He proceeded to let me know it was not Mt. Kilimanjaro, Mt. Everest, or anything close to that. He was simply hoping to climb Mt. L.A. Fitness. With a big smile on his face and speaking from the heart, he shared that he wanted to go the gym and work through physical and mental obstacles, push some weights, and, if possible, get some cardio in. Not being able to train as hard or with the same intensity he was used to was a challenge in and of itself, but it would certainly not be an obstacle he didn't choose to overcome.

Doug is always one to look at the cup half full instead of half empty, and with this in mind, he would always close the day out by saying, "Today was a good day." It didn't matter how difficult, challenging, or exhausting the day may have been, he was grateful for the privilege of living it out. That evening as we gathered in the family room to reflect on our day and have communion together, Doug reminded us that God wanted to turn not just our crisis but everyone else's crises into victories. We just needed to allow God to work and not get in His way. Then Doug went on to say, "Today was a good day, but some days are better good days, and today was a better good day." I had tears of joy in my eyes.

My husband, who had an uncomfortable line running through his arm and into his heart, whose body was receiving a strong poison to kill the cancer cells, and who was putting up with me and my rules of a restricted diet and gross-tasting protocols, dealing with occasional nausea, and dependent on me to help him in many humbling ways, instead of being angry, chose to tell us, "It was a better good day." He demonstrated to Ashley, Mom, and me what champions were made of. With God on his side, no matter the outcome, his joy would not be taken, period! The joy of the Lord was truly his strength. (See Psalm 28:7.)

THE EAGLE IS BALDING

During one of our hospital appointments, I met a patient that told me she had lost all of her body hair, including nose hairs, five days into her chemo treatment. I had mentally prepared myself for the possibility, but spoke life into Doug's body and prayed against it. With each passing day, I believed that the lack of hair loss was a wink from heaven. I guess it was, as it could have happened sooner.

At the end of June, I began to notice hair in the tub after Doug's baths or showers. I would clean it up and not say a word to him, processing if this was the start of his hairless season due to the chemotherapy treatments. I recall making the bed in the mornings and finding hair there, too.

With each day that passed, I found more hair in the tub and in the bedding. I would wait until he left for work and then strip the bed, take the sheets outside to shake as much of the body hair off as possible and then wash them in hopes they would all come off. For about five days, I was washing our bedding every day without him knowing, until one day, he said, "Honey, am I losing my hair?" Oh, to be able to describe the look on my face. "Yes," I replied, not wanting to draw much attention to it. Then I heard him say, "Bummers, my hair is everywhere. I'm sorry."

Finally, there were no more undercover cleaning missions. I had been trying to protect him from something he could probably care less about. I am quite sure that for females, this would be a different story. Oftentimes, our hair is a part of our personality and most of us like styling it, coloring it, and getting creative with our hairdos during different stages in our lives.

Hair loss is a sad reality for many cancer patients. When you are walking through a battle of this sort, it is not about vanity; it's about appreciating the little things in life. Doug was a trooper and not scared to face himself in the mirror; I, on the other hand, loved his hair and wanted it to stay right where it was.

Yes, I could have been honest with him from the beginning. Everyone's story is different and what drives us to make those decisions at the time depends on many circumstances. Perhaps I was in denial, wanting to believe he would not have to go through that, or perhaps I just wanted to protect him from realizing the extra work it took to clean up the results of the hair loss. In fact, I recall sweeping the hairs off the tile in the bathroom and running the vacuum cleaner in our bedroom daily as well. It's not that he had tons of hair, but dark hairs on light tile are noticeable, and I just preferred to have everything as clean as possible. One thing for sure is that the balding was evidence that he was in the middle of a war with cancer.

A FULL DAY AHEAD

It was well after midnight on July third when my tired body crawled into bed. Before taking part in the typical holiday celebrations on the following day, which often include family barbecues, pool time, people enjoying the day at parks and beaches, and the spectacular displays of fireworks that close out the evening in just about every community in the U.S., we had chosen to take part in a prayer gathering for our nation. Ashley was on the worship team, so she and I needed to be at the church extra early. Because Doug was scheduled to be the speaker and set the tone for this gathering of prayer leaders and pastors of the greater Houston area, we decided to go in separate cars, giving Doug the chance to sleep in.

After only a couple hours of sleep, Doug who had yet to go to sleep, woke me up to share a revelation he had. Oh, the joys of having a night owl for a husband! Even a diagnosis of cancer did not slow this man down.

He jokingly, but seriously said, "Honey, wake up, wake up! The eagle is balding." I shot up in bed, concerned. *What on earth is going on? Is he okay? Did he hurt himself? But then again, why is he full of joy? What time is it?* Dazed, propped up on my arms, I stared at him. My arms just wanted to give out and allow me to lie back down. "Honey, seriously, the eagle is balding!" I could not believe it. I was physically tired and Doug was almost dancing around our bed with excitement that he was going bald— something I already knew.

DOUG SHARES A REVELATION

Then suddenly, as I came fully alert and decided to embrace whatever it was he was experiencing, he began to share his heart. Eagles have incredible eyesight because they have a second fovea or depression in the retina of their eyes, which allows them to see very small details from great distances. It is said that they are able to spot an object as small as a rabbit from up to two miles away. They also have three eyelids, one which is clear and can be shut for protection while not inhibiting their ability to see.

Some say there is no creature that can stare at the sun without going blind; others say the extra eyelid on the eagle allows it to look into the sun without harm. Regardless, when feeling weak and weary, eagles will soar toward the sun, even above the storms and threatening clouds, to rejuvenate themselves. This is what Scripture speaks of when it says, *"But those who wait on the LORD shall renew their strength; they shall mount up with wings like eagles, they shall run and not be weary, they shall walk and not faint"* (Isaiah 40:31).

The Lord had reminded Doug that America's national bird is the bald eagle. God began to minister to Doug's heart about the condition of our nation at that time, disheartened and weakened. Initially, the joke was about him losing his hair, but as God began to give him a download, that quickly changed. The bald eagle, to America, actually represents strength and courage.

This would be another reminder that our life experiences become part of our life messages, which are bigger than ourselves—messages beyond the circumstances we've been through. They are a reminder that we are overcomers by the blood of the Lamb and the word of our testimony. (See Revelation 12:11.) Doug passionately related the importance of the eagle in America, except he added that when we are weak and weary, we must not give in, but shoot straight for the brightness of the Son. He also cited Hebrews 12:2, fixing our eyes on Jesus, *"the author and finisher of our faith."*

"THIS EAGLE WILL RENEW ITS STRENGTH"

As Doug finished sharing, he stared straight into my eyes with confidence and a smile on his face and said, "The eagle is balding, but this eagle will renew its strength, I shall run and not be weary, I shall walk and not faint as I wait on the Lord, and I will soar towards the Son, Jesus, the author and finisher of my faith."

I had gotten a Bible study in the middle of the night and he clearly wanted me to have as much joy as he did over every bit of his download. How could I possibly go back to sleep after that?

Morning came and armed with my Bible and a cup of coffee, we were off to the prayer gathering. It was a powerful way to start our Independence Day celebration. Doug gave such an encouraging word. He reminded us that we were a generation that needed strength to come into our destiny and only the brightness of His presence would reveal the greater reality and greater authority that God wields. Doug reminded us that when we fix our eyes on Jesus, we can soar above our weakness and renew our strength to fulfill God's call and destiny in our lives and nation. He closed by reminding us that we should not be informed only by what we saw and heard on the news, nor let the circumstances around us dictate who we are. God has the final word. *Who would we believe?* He stated with a firm voice, "I choose to believe the Word of the Lord. He never waivers. He is the same yesterday, today, and forever."

Shortly after leaving the prayer gathering, we received numerous encouraging messages from people who were touched by the Word in season. One person wrote to tell us that the banner on the front of the *Houston Chronicle* says, "Long live the bald eagle." Our national symbol is on the rebound. The actual article on the inside read, "A nation unites to save the bald eagles." How amazing is this in light of Doug's teaching on "The Eagle Is Balding." Our God is so good. In addition, Doug had received texts and emails from various spiritual sons, all of whom had separately sent him the following Scripture: *"But to you who fear My name the Sun of Righteousness shall arise with healing in His wings"* (Malachi 4:2).

At times, when Doug feels tired and overwhelmed, he quotes David Livingstone, a missionary from the 1800s: "Why is it that when an earthly king commissions us we consider it an honor, but when commissioned by the Heavenly King, we consider it a sacrifice?" Doug adds, "It is not a sacrifice to be a part of the Lord's service; it's truly an honor and privilege!"

THIS EAGLE SOARED WITH HOPE

With that being said, it was a great Fourth of July. Our family had the privilege of having Ashley serve on the worship team, Doug shared and led us in prayer, and I was blessed to gather with others to worship and pray for our nation. It was a good day—in fact, it was a better good day. My eagle may have been balding, but he was soaring with hope because his trust was in the Lord. I recall telling him, "Douglas, you may become bald by tomorrow, but I know you will continue to soar to the Son, from where your strength comes from; you will soar like never before, with greater strength, power, anointing, and grace. I love you, my cancer-beating prince; with or without hair, you will always have my heart."

The morning of July fifth came around and with it a man who didn't complain about the morning ritual of healthy drinks and eats. After Doug's devotion time, he asked me to follow him to the front of the house and take a photo of him. He posed in front of the door and said, "I am ready for special duty, Sir!" What did he mean? He then proceeded to share that he was talking to God. He had his weapons of warfare in hand: an appeal to heaven for God's intervention in his spirit; his heart and prayers for awakening and revival; and his thanks to God, who always leads us to victory and triumph.

Doug had a wedding to officiate that afternoon. It was evident that his hair was a bit patchy and not as full as it once was. He asked me if he should shave it to eliminate the trail it would leave throughout the house. I suggested he wait until after the wedding, and he agreed. He was careful not to touch it much, for strands of it would easily come out in his hands.

Before leaving the house, he reminded me of the importance of this day for the bride, groom, and their family and friends. He reminded me that God did not do this to him, so it didn't belong to him, and it should not be about him or us for that matter. With that being said, if anyone asked us how we were doing, we were to say "good" and redirect the conversation back to the joy of the moment we were all privileged to be witnessing. Doug wanted to make sure that he didn't become the center of attention, for even a moment. That was not the place or time to discuss anything about cancer or anything Stringer. It was a time of celebration for the beautiful young couple and their family, and I would honor his request.

TIME FOR A BUZZ CUT

After returning home, we had one mission in mind: get that head shaved. We chose a buzz cut instead of shaving it off completely. I guess I wanted to see the transition. Looking back now, I realize how blessed I am, as Doug wanted to save me the trouble of cleaning up even the little hairs that fell from his head, which would eventually end up all over the place. But I wanted a day to experience the transition to bald, hence the buzz cut.

As the night came to a close and our family gathered for our nightly time of reflection, prayer, and communion, Doug shared that, "It is unavoidable that obstacles, hardships, distractions, and trials will confront believers and tempt us to doubt God's faithfulness. Challenges and adversities are only temporary obstacles filled with opportunities of a greater testimony because we serve a faithful and great God. He cares because extravagant is His love towards us."

Doug was always teaching us, growing us, and stretching us to think beyond our circumstances. Negativity was not allowed, nor was it even an option. He finished by saying, "I agree with King David, 'I've never seen the righteous forsaken...' Our God is awesome and mighty and His love never fails."

If ever there were moments of doubt or sadness, during our daily communion time, the negative feelings would always be washed away. God's Word does that. Having a leader who reminds you of His Word and demonstrates it to you firsthand through his actions and words is an undeniable and powerful witness to the power of truth.

Out of Doug's mouth came the following on a regular basis: "Thank You, Abba, for Your Father's embrace, encouragement, assurance, affirmation, strength, wisdom, guidance, and abounding grace to stay the course, fixing our eyes on You." He would say that while praying before our meals, or as we walked into hospitals, not for his care, but to visit others who we wanted to support and pray for, or out of the blue while driving to a destination to serve. Thanksgiving was and is always on his lips.

With this active demonstration of appreciation, to this day, he has shown us how to live with a grateful heart. I am even more grateful that Ashley has had the greatest of role models in walking out our faith and witnessing the power of prayer. She has seen firsthand what having a warrior of the King to lead the house looks like and she was being shown a standard of qualities that she could desire in the husband she would someday marry.

In the 2010 movie, *The Voyage of the Dawn Treader*, based on the book by C. S. Lewis, one character says, "Hardships often prepare ordinary people for an extraordinary destiny." I chose to believe that on the other side of this journey, we were going to live out an extraordinary destiny, if we kept our eyes on our destination.

8

THE FRIEND FACTOR

Living in a city with over six million people, including the surrounding areas, what is the probability that we would run into someone we knew at MDA? Moreover, what is the probability that co-laborers and pastors would be patients at the same time Doug was scheduled at the hospital? With God, there are no coincidences. He is all-knowing and a God of providence. I found it amazing, however, that on at least eight occasions that we were scheduled at the hospital, we ran into others we knew who were either receiving treatment or having a battery of tests done.

> WITH GOD, THERE ARE NO COINCIDENCES.
> HE IS ALL-KNOWING AND A GOD OF PROVIDENCE.

On one such occasion, we were able to visit with Pastors Dusty and Mary Kemp of New Life Church, who were also in between various appointments. The Kemps had been such a great inspiration, encouragement, and source of wisdom throughout the battle and had graciously clued us in on the process. We loved the opportunity to talk as friends and share His revelation outside of a formal event or conference. Our time to pray for one another was icing on the cake. In the midst of it all, we prayed for awakening and revival!

Looking back on that day, before me stood two well-respected pastors in the city of Houston who had labored together for decades, serving Houstonians and beyond. They had been part of services where people who were hungry for God's presence were healed of all kinds of infirmities and made whole spiritually and emotionally. These men had worshipped and taken communion together many a time. Yet at that moment, Doug and Dusty had patient identification bracelets on their wrists; they were on the opposite side of the fence, and both still testifying to the goodness of our God. Neither one was there on a pastoral visit for a member of their congregation, ministry partner, or friend; they were simply patients. Not one of them, but both of them. How was it that one and the other were on a journey that included pain, inconvenience, emotional and financial challenges, new levels of trust in God, and so much more? It was all because of a cancer diagnosis.

RECEIVING A NEW MISSION FIELD

Doug and Dusty had an all-access pass to a new mission field. Not that they didn't before; as pastors, they both made many visits at all hours of the day or night to be with patients in their times of need. But this time, they had a new level of authority or credibility that came with the experience of being patients themselves. Doug often says, "This was a ministry we didn't ask for, but it was a ministry nonetheless." He says "we" because as a married couple, we are partners, co-laborers. We often make hospital or home visits together and when we can't, we lend each other the time away from family to serve those with greater needs.

There were many friends who would call and ask if Doug would meet them or their loved ones or friends for a time of prayer and encouragement. So in between doctor's appointments and tests, we would find ourselves in one of the hospital's many lobbies or patient rooms, experiencing special times of fellowship. We would laugh a bit, reminisce, and talk about the future and what we were all going to do when the season of battling cancer was over. We dreamt together, reassured one another, and always prayed for each other and the many who had needs in the hospital and around the globe.

We always meant what we prayed and believed with our hearts that healing could and would come. Ultimately, one way or another, our faith led us to believing that we would find our healing. Hebrews 11:1 says, *"Now faith is the substance of things hoped for, the evidence of things not seen."* I admit that in the natural, there were times when our friends looked like they were holding on for their lives. This did not deter our prayers, which are always driven by faith. If we did not hold on to hope, specifically the hope of glory, in many cases, we would have been defeated quickly.

Our hearts could believe, but our minds would easily doubt because of the evidence before us. There were a few times when we prayed with people who looked like death was knocking at their door. At times, death may knock, but it doesn't mean we have to answer. I have seen documentaries of some who, as they say, "cheated death" and I have read testimonies of some who have been declared dead and yet live today. God has the ultimate say.

Not everyone's story will be the same. I don't know why some live and others enter the portals of eternity sooner than expected, but I do know that God is faithful. I trust Him and I will choose to pray with faith that moves mountains. If in the natural I am discouraged by what I see and let my mind rule my heart, then it is easy to feel like I've fallen into a pit that I cannot climb out of. I will let my heart rule over my mind because that is where Jesus dwells.

> AT TIMES, DEATH MAY KNOCK, BUT IT DOESN'T MEAN WE HAVE TO ANSWER. GOD HAS THE ULTIMATE SAY.

ASHLEY PENS "SAVE THE DAY"

There is a song our daughter wrote when she was thirteen years old that made it on her first EP (extended play record). It's called "Save the Day" and the lyrics go like this:

Sometimes we go through things

We just don't understand, oh just

To let go and be safe in Your hands.

I'm taking one step at a time.

With You on my side everything will be alright.

I'm learning to breathe and fly.

No more pain or bruises, I'm flying high.

When I close my eyes, the light starts coming.

The fog fades away,

That's when I can see Your face.

No matter the fire, I will walk right through it.

My Hero will save

The day, because He is not far away.

I want to shout about how Your love rescued me.

Oh and how You set the captives free.

This world will always try to pull You down.

But there is One name that will always be around.

Say His name.

The meaning behind the lyrics is deep and powerful and was perfect during our season of battling cancer. Part of the process of healing for us was learning to let go and trust that no matter what the circumstance was, we would be safe in the hands of God. The song reminded us that when we closed our eyes, we could focus on God and not be distracted with all the negative sights or noise pollution that surrounded us. The fog would fade and His presence would reign, which in turn brought peace.

We had to be intentional about not allowing the inevitable hits to leave deep scars. And with the assurance of His love, we were truly free and could get through even the toughest times. By no means am I saying these times were tearless; I am just stating that we got through them because of His love and abounding grace.

As of the publishing of this book, there were people we prayed for who had every medical statistic against them and a low survival rate, yet they are still with us, appreciating every day, testifying to God's goodness, and making a difference in the world. With a heavy heart, I must mention that there were others, true champions and mighty kingdom warriors, who were called home to be with Him.

For those of us who call upon the name of the Lord, death is nothing to fear. Second Corinthians 5:8 (TPT) says, *"We live with a joyful confidence, yet at the same time we take delight in the thought of leaving our bodies behind to be at home with the Lord.*" It is, however, a time of great mourning for those who have lost their special someone, resting only in the confidence that we will see each other again in our eternal home and in the presence of God.

Having talked to some patients and thinking of our own story, it is not that we wouldn't at times just want to throw in the towel and say, "I am done," with regard to anything. But it was the thought of not wanting to leave the family behind that would often be the bigger struggle. A mother who had young children would want to be able to guide and teach them as they grew. A father would want to walk his daughter down the aisle on her wedding day or be there for his kids' graduation celebrations. Thoughts of that kind led to tears. Yet when you trust in God, even those very emotional moments ultimately find peace because the Giver of all peace brings comfort to those who mourn.

PRE-TREATMENT FORMALITIES

There were many times early on when Doug was asked about the cancer diagnosis and his response was almost always the same. "I have to focus on what I am supposed to do. I know my vision, I know what God wants us to do, and I know there are people we are supposed to reach. I just don't feel like our time is up, so that is what we focus on. We keep our vision on our destination rather than on what we are going through."

Doug was self-motivated and I believe much of the motivation was inspired from his intimate encounters with the Lord. He took time to hear God's voice and then followed His lead. One of the best decisions we could have made was to take communion prior to the start of each chemotherapy treatment. This was a non-negotiable, something he knew would bring our family peace and keep us in sync with each other, but mostly with God. He also determined that we would always have an attitude of gratitude, no matter what.

After checking in and being assigned a bed and private room in the infusion area of the hospital, we would meet our nurse for the day. Doug always thanked them in advance for all they would be doing, explaining our pre-treatment Stringer family ritual, which included a time of worship, prayer, and communion prior to having the infusion start, always inviting the medical staff to take part. All but one of the nurses throughout the course of our treatment joined us during the communion portion. The nurses set up the IV and medications, going in and out of Doug's room, as they had other patients to tend to as well.

With smiles on their faces, each one stopped to join in as we prayed and took communion. Some commented on how blessed they were to be a part of our special time, recognizing that there was One above all who was overseeing the process. All of the assigned staff thanked us for allowing them to be a part of the intimate experience.

With every infusion, different friends and co-laborers joined us in setting the atmosphere, bringing peace into the room and in our hearts. Pastor Mike May, who is also a videographer and producer, was capturing our every moment with the intent of producing short videos that would encourage others and eventually become a documentary of our journey. Throughout the course of writing this book, I took the time to again watch some of the short takes. It was hard to not do so without being moved deeply, experiencing a plethora of emotions that powerfully touched me in exuberant measures. They will always serve as reminders of God's faithfulness along the way. No matter what tomorrow holds, I will recall the landmark moments when God showed Himself faithful and trustworthy, allowing us to experience miracles and breakthroughs throughout our journey.

TIME FOR ROUND TWO

Before starting the second round of chemotherapy, I recall looking at the clock, noting the potential start time. I glanced at the room full of family and friends, which included a now-bald Ruben. He had shaved his head as a way of standing with Doug during this season and told Doug that the bald eagles were rising and fixing their eyes on the Son.

Each person was holding their communion cup, with eyes beginning to close as Doug began to pray out loud, "We speak life and we thank You that even as they put in the R-CHOP and all the other stuff that is going into my body, this is Your temple and Your blood cleanses us, purges us and also purifies us. This is Your temple, Lord. We are asking that as it goes in, that it will kill what needs to be killed, destroying the cancer. The big C is Jesus Christ. You are our Healer, You are Jehovah Rapha, You are the Healer, and are the Great Physician. We thank You for all the great medical staff at MD Anderson and we thank You for the wisdom and the heart that You have given to them and so many. We receive that love, Lord, and that sensitivity. Now we are asking You, Great Physician, that as You oversee this whole process, that what goes into my body will only kill what needs to be killed and You would speak life and give life, because life is in Your blood, in Jesus's name."

With prayers like that coming from the patient himself, how could I not experience a peace that surpasses all understanding? The activist Corrie ten Boom once said, "Is prayer your steering wheel or your spare tire?" Many of us find ourselves remembering to pray when we are in a desperate situation. We pray passionate and heartfelt prayers that we are hoping will touch the heart of God. In our brokenness, we often get lost in desperate prayer and lose track of time. But for many of us, in our season of rest, joy, health, and financial peace, we totally embrace the "spare tire prayer tactic," praying a quick minute or two and calling it a day. It is during this time that we rarely wash our mind with the Word of God, nor spend time worshipping Him, simply for who He is.

I would like to think that prayer has been our steering wheel, with the difference being that in this season, we were in a fierce storm and the view in front of us was very limited at times. Imagine struggling to see because of a downpour of rain. You are leaning forward as close as you can to the steering wheel, hoping for a better view of the road ahead, windshield wipers going full speed. Your grip on the steering wheel is so tight, your palms are clammy and sweaty. That was me!

I recall someone asking Doug how he could pray for healing in others if he himself had a big need. They questioned why God had not healed him yet and how he could actually believe that God could heal others. I'll never forget part of his response, "Our circumstance doesn't change who God is, but God can change our circumstance. God is the same yesterday, today, and forever! He is more than able and God's timing is always perfect." Wow, what a profound and penetrating statement.

> OUR CIRCUMSTANCE DOESN'T CHANGE WHO GOD IS, BUT GOD CAN CHANGE OUR CIRCUMSTANCE. HE IS MORE THAN ABLE AND GOD'S TIMING IS ALWAYS PERFECT. —DOUG

God was in control and Doug had no doubt about it. God is still in the healing business. Sometimes our healing comes on earth and others times it comes in heaven.

MANY WINKS FROM HEAVEN

Throughout our journey, God sent us many winks from heaven from some of His earthly angels; dear friends who dropped off gifts, balloons, cards, and all kinds of blessings, including coffee to our home or ministry office. On one occasion, some ladies all wore green to symbolize life and put up blue ribbons on our rocking chair and elsewhere to represent living water. One of the gifts was a prayer cloth that the children of Harvest Home Orphanage in Hyderabad, India, had prayed over and sent as a reminder that people from all over the globe were praying in agreement for Doug's healing.

I served on the board that supports this and other orphanages in India. Ashley was only six years old when she and I made our first trip to serve them. We fell in love with the children and are able to communicate with them often through FaceTime and social media. The prayer cloth was a meaningful and sentimental gift that we still treasure.

Doug was very moved by our friends' actions and choked up when he saw the abundance of love as he began to read the many notes that were forwarded to us. Michael W. Smith has a song lyric that resonates within us: "Friends are friends forever if the Lord is the Lord of them." We are grateful for lifetime friends, for their generous hearts, unfailing prayers, and unselfish love. I recall feeling a tad awkward and very humbled, as we enjoy giving more than receiving.

It was a new experience for me to receive in every way at this level, but one that brought perspective and taught me more life lessons. God reminded me that He would provide, even in the littlest of things. He used close friends to manifest His love on a regular basis. I know God multiplies every seed sown in love, and our prayers were that He would return many times over the kind gestures shown to us by the many who helped us along the way, help that made a significant difference impacting my faith and proving His word true.

John 15:13 says, *"Greater love has no one than this, than to lay down one's life for his friends."* We truly experienced the love, generosity, and prayers of friends, which thrusted us forward in faith and with peace.

PILLOWS OF PEACE

One of the gifts we received is what we began to call the pillow of peace. Virginia Miniel Savala, the mother of Emily Zavala, a Somebody Cares staff member, would write Scriptures on pillows for her family. Emily's sister, Patricia Laredo, continued this precious tradition and wrote Scriptures on pillows for her own daughters so they could literally rest on the Word of God. When Patricia heard about Doug's cancer trial, she created one of the most beautiful gifts we had ever received, our very own pillow of peace. Her daughter, Leah Laredo Grafton, brought it to our home and shared that she still sleeps on the pillow her mom made for her long ago.

We posted a photo of the pillow, adorned with Scriptures that spoke life, healing, and hope, all written in bright-colored sharpies. The request for these comfy pieces of art started coming in from all over the country and around the globe. People battling cancer, depression, and other medical challenges were emailing us, asking if we could send one to them, a friend, or a family member in need of encouragement. Leah noticed the requests that were posted on my social media page and immediately responded. With the help of her three sisters, they purchased and created more pillows for us to give away. It got to the point where we could not create them fast enough. A few of my friends heard of the need and met me at a local pizza parlor, each one with pillows and bibles in tow. We ordered pizzas, brought our kids, and went to town creating each unique pillow. Our table was our workstation. We wrote Scriptures on them and prayed for the people who would receive the colorful, comforting, and motivating gifts, as well as their families.

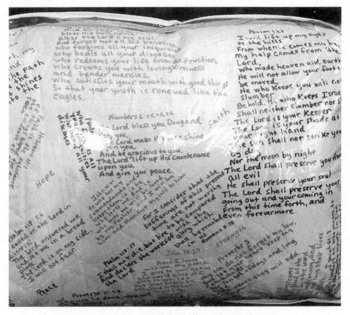

Patricia Laredo created this pillow of peace for Doug.

While in the restaurant, people's curiosity was piqued and many began to ask what we were doing. As we shared, customers and employees in the restaurant began to encourage us and thank us for our hearts to serve others, some even stopping to pray for the pillow recipients. A few people asked if they could borrow the idea and create them as well. We let them know it was not our idea—we were just paying it forward. This would happen in every public place we gathered to create the pillows, opening many doors for opportunities to share God's love.

The pillow of peace movement began with a praying grand-mother who wanted the Word of God to be with her family, even in their rest. Who would have thought that this would impact so many in such a positive way? Ashley, Doug, and I delivered many pillows to people in hospitals throughout Houston and surrounding areas. Reflecting on that season, we truly embraced the new ministry assignment the Lord had given us. Our family visited many who were hospitalized, worshipped with them, prayed, and, in some cases, took communion with them. This became a more regular part of our lives and is true still today. I wish I could tell you the need has not been as great, but for some reason, we have had an increase in the number of people we know who have since been diagnosed with cancer or have had a need for a medical miracle. As often as time permits, we visit them in their time of need and, at the very least, we call to pray with them over the phone.

Doug was in the middle of his own trial, but it didn't stop him from serving others and bringing them the hope that comes from washing our minds with the Word of God. With the pillows, it was hope that they could literally rest on. As Doug would remind us every time we left a pastoral care visit, "This was a ministry we did not ask for, but it was a ministry nonetheless." Pastoral care visits have and will always be a part of what we do, but with the new challenge, each visit is a reminder that we have a new level of authority and relatability to those we were visiting and interceding for.

Because of the time it takes to create each pillow, we were grateful for the many friends, including homeschool groups, who chose to sow of their time and resources to purchase and design the pillows that were shipped across the country. The joy that people reflected is a priceless memory. As some looked at their gift and read many of the Scriptures aloud, tears would stream down their faces as they declared their trust in God. Some even thanked God for the medical challenges they found themselves in as they too felt it was an opportunity to testify of His goodness. These patients would choose to praise Him in the midst of their storm. This was a heartwarming experience that brought plenty of tears to our eyes.

We received cards from all over, expressing gratitude that we would take the time to send such a symbolic gift. We also received photos of patients sleeping on their pillows. I hear Doug share often that obedience is the highest form of worship and that we will never know until we enter the portals of eternity the depth and width of the impact we have made in people's lives. I believe God showed us a small glimpse through the many people who received these pillows.

The pillow of peace creator, who was a praying and loving grandmother, could not have imagined what would become of her simple obedience to fashion an atmosphere of peace for her kids that would someday touch people beyond her reach and generation. I am grateful to her family for sharing the love of Christ through the pillows of peace with us. If this resonates with you, pick up your sharpies, pray about the Scriptures, and create your own "best present ever." These are not only for people who are sick or weary, but for anyone you love or want to share God's love with. The pillow is another way for some to pray the Scriptures and a reminder that we can run the race before us with peace that surpasses all understanding. No matter what the outcome in any situation, if we give freely, lovingly, deeply, and compassionately, God wins, and we are all the better for it.

GOD HEARS US WHEN WE SEEK HIM, FREES US FROM OUR FEARS, AND DELIVERS THE RIGHTEOUS FROM THEIR TROUBLES.

Psalm 34, titled "The Happiness of Those Who Trust in God," begins, *I will bless the* LORD *at all times.*" This psalm by King David, which is among the verses on our pillow, says God hears us when we seek Him, frees us from our fears, and delivers the righteous from their troubles. When you are hurting, Scriptures like this can restore hope and give rest. There is power in the Word of God and it truly changes the game. For our family, it sustains us through the roughest of storms.

A WORD OF ENCOURAGEMENT

Early in our journey, I read about the side effects of the medication Doug would be receiving to kill the cancer in his body. Exhausted, I sat in front of the computer, clicking from article to article. Some included photos and testimonies of family members of patients. I recall saying, "Great, so according to this, my husband can survive cancer, but he might have heart issues and a possible heart attack?" At the time, it was too much reality too quickly. Reading such information qualified as one of the most painful and emotional experiences I had in the early days. The more I read, the more my heart ached.

I called my cousin, Elsa Huerta, who has been my mentor. She has encouraged me when I was at my lowest, always directing me to the Lord and showing me His love in tangible ways. God used her powerfully during this season as she infused me with specific, life-giving Scriptures exactly when I needed them. Elsa was like an archer, shooting an arrow at a small target and hitting the mark every time. She could do this because of her intimate relationship with God. When I needed a shoulder to cry on, she inspired my spirit with the Word of God, never letting me stay depressed and making sure negative thoughts were buried and gone.

Doug says everyone needs a true friend who will speak truth in love seasoned with grace, someone who will speak life and strengthen you in God's Word, someone who you can count on to always be honest with you, even when you don't want to hear it. A friend never gives up on you, even when death knocks on your door.

We all need friends who remind us not to let our circumstances dictate who we are, but to remember who we are in Christ. Such friends will encourage us to bring our mind and body in subjection to the spirit of God, and then make sure we're not just talking a good game, but walking it out. I was blessed to have a handful of friends that I could count on who made sure I read the Word, prayed the Word, and lived the Word.

A real friend will also remind us that adversities are opportunities for us to fix our eyes on the Lord, the author and finisher of our faith. (See Hebrews 12:2.) Doug has said, "The true character of an individual is revealed and magnified most during times of crisis, change, and challenge." My foundation was solid, but at times, my structure felt weak and compromised. The emotional and physical blows took a toll on me.

> SURROUND YOURSELF WITH FRIENDS WHO ARE STRONG IN THE LORD, WHO WILL LIFT YOU UP—AS AARON AND HUR DID FOR MOSES—IN YOUR TIME OF WEAKNESS.

Surround yourself with friends who are strong in the Lord, who will lift you up—as Aaron and Hur did for Moses—in your time of weakness.

Doug also says, "To fight the battles of this life in our own strength is to invite discouragement, eventual failure, and defeat. When we are compromising in our walk with God, we will be ineffective in our witness and work for God."

9

DOUG RUNS THE ROCKY STEPS

It was a beautiful day in mid-August when Doug and I headed for the airport to take part in a ministry assignment. We were both excited to be participating in it. While business as usual, it held an added dose of gratitude for all the Lord had done and was doing in and through us. This is what we lived for, to see lives changed and the love of the Lord shared everywhere we went. Doug had determined to not let cancer take his joy away, no matter what!

As we readied to board our flight, I realized people were staring. For a moment, I wondered what they were looking at. *Did I have a tag hanging somewhere? Had I sat on something that left a stain on my pants?* Then Doug asked me a question. As I turned to respond, it hit me. I understood what some where thinking and maybe saying to one another. They weren't staring at me. They were fixated on the man standing next to me, who was thin, bald, and wearing a surgical mask.

People probably thought he was a cancer patient, or at the very least, a sick person. I was used to Doug wearing the mask so it didn't faze me. It was simply part of the protocol.

I've been guilty of doing the same thing, noticing people who wore the same mask, who looked weak and sick. I always tried not to stare, but at times, I probably did. I was intentional about smiling, making eye contact, and when possible and appropriate, engaging them in conversation.

It's possible that people were saying things like, "Poor guy," or maybe, "Let's pray for him." And maybe, someone shared with his travel mate, "I am so grateful I have my health today." I'll never know and it doesn't really matter. As with other experiences on our journey, it was one I learned from and made me grow. I developed perspective, empathy, and compassion for the many who had gone before us and those who were yet to walk in our shoes.

One of the challenges of being a parent of a young child is teaching them when to speak and when to be quiet. Another is when to ask us a question. Let's face it, some questions are better asked and answered in private.

As we waited to board our flight, a little boy said loudly, "What's wrong with him? Is that man sick, Daddy?" I can smile at this now, but I recall feeling awkward for the parents. The mom reacted by slapping the boy's hand, telling him to be quiet. I felt badly for the boy. He didn't know any better. He just asked an honest and innocent question out loud. Neither parent answered him, so the boy asked again. Finally, the mom said, "I don't know. Maybe." I gave them a smile.

I don't know if Doug even heard him, as we have never talked about it. Doug was returning emails on his phone, taking advantage of the cell service prior to takeoff. If we hadn't boarded right after this incident, I might have gone over and talked to him and his parents for a bit, letting the boy know that Doug was just trying to keep the germ monsters away. Once seated, more passengers stared as they walked down the aisle to their seats. There were also smiles and even a few winks.

Many times, Doug and I have gone to the airport to pick up pastors, friends, and even friends of friends who had flown to Houston to receive treatment at MD Anderson. When possible, we provided transportation for them, sat with them during treatments, or visited during hospital stays, since many didn't have family or friends in Houston. Sometimes, I picked up people I'd never met who were too weak to walk from the airplane through the airport and to the waiting car. Our first meeting was when an escort wheeled them to our car in the passenger pickup area. Some were too nauseous to talk, so the only sound during the drive to the hospital was soft worship music in the background.

It's hard to describe what I've seen some patients and their families go through. I can't fathom what all the hospital staff witnesses—everything imaginable and even unimaginable. I've always respected those in the medical field, but because of our experiences, I've gained a new, higher level of regard for these heroes who give not just physically but emotionally too.

READY TO SERVE...AND RUN

We landed in Philadelphia feeling good and ready to serve. We were excited to join Ross and Ruth Willard, who were hosting a "Kings and Priests" gathering at a church over an hour-and-a-half west, in Lancaster, Pennsylvania. While driving through Philadelphia along Interstate 76, we admired the beauty of the city, the bridges, the Schuylkill River, and much more. Suddenly, we saw the Philadelphia Museum of Art across the river and were told about the Rocky Statue at the top of the Ben Franklin Parkway in Center City. Doug said, "Maybe we can make time to visit the art museum before we leave. I could run by the Flags of the Nations, interceding for the countries represented, then run the steps like Sylvester Stallone did in the movie *Rocky*."

When we minister in cities throughout the world, we rarely have opportunities to see the historic sites or landmarks. When possible, we've booked ourselves an extra day, but time doesn't usually permit it. Returning home or to our next assignment takes precedence.

I thought it was a great idea and encouraged him to do it. I even said I'd do it with him, sure I could own up to what I was committing, unlike the healthy smoothies that I failed to drink because of the unpleasant taste.

It was all but done! I determined to make time in our schedule for the tourist attraction, do what his heart wanted to do, and witness the joy it would bring him.

Throughout the conference, we were encouraged as we heard other speakers preach. I believe others were inspired when Doug preached. I know I was. He may have looked a little weathered, but was energetic and passionate as he taught and shared God's love. I knew that the prayer coverage we were receiving played a significant part in how Doug was responding.

During the conference, we made new friends, met co-laborers in ministry, and shared the gospel with those in attendance and beyond. Doug never misses an opportunity to share the good news with those whose paths he crosses. He believes these encounters are divine appointments. When the conference ended, we moved to a hotel near the airport. This allowed us to sleep in a bit and not contend with traffic. Often, when we have a rental car, we return it the night before and take the hotel shuttle to the airport, saving us money and time on the day of departure.

We enjoyed a late dinner in the hotel restaurant prior to returning the rental car. I talked about how excited I was that we were going to run the *Rocky* steps the next morning. I was cheering Doug on when the waiter overheard our conversation. He told us that the art museum was on many people's bucket lists of places to visit in Philly.

Early in our conversation, Doug asked our waiter if there was anything he could pray about for him. There weren't many customers in the restaurant, which allowed us to spend more time interacting. Doug told about his cancer journey. The short-sleeve shirt Doug wore made it obvious he had a medical device attached to his arm. He then shared how he maintained peace in the midst of the storm because of his faith. That intrigued the waiter and led to more dialogue.

WAITER OFFERS SOME ADVICE

By this time, the waiter learned from Doug about his desire to jog the path of the various nations' flags, run up the *Rocky* steps, and raise his arms in victory like Stallone did. The waiter suggested we drive over instead of taking the train or a cab. He gave us directions for getting there easily to avoid traffic and told us where to park.

The waiter was in awe of Doug's determination to run, despite being a cancer patient in the midst of treatment with a PICC line attached to his body. At the same time, he was thrilled for us. I think that witnessing our joy and desire to press toward our goals brought him hope and encouragement in the midst of his personal trials. By the end of our meal, he was cheering us on. He made Doug promise to leave word if he accomplished the goal and how it went.

Once settled into our hotel room, I set aside the clothes for our jog and the clothes we would change into for our flight home. I calculated how much time we needed for the jog and run up the steps, hotel checkout, return of the rental car, and making it to the airport in time for our flight home. I told Doug what time the alarm would wake us in the morning. I asked if he agreed with that time, but didn't get a response. I looked at him, but he just gave me "a look." I knew that look, but wasn't sure if I was interpreting it correctly.

By this time, with food in our bellies, he was ready to settle down and recuperate from the busy day we'd had. We still had to flush his lines and take care of the daily medical protocol. Time was escaping us. We were tired and on a downward spiral.

Doug went about his business, taking a shower, packing, and spending some time returning emails and a few phone calls. I eventually suggested we call it a night since we had an early morning adventure. Once again, I asked if he agreed with the wakeup time. This time, he said, "Maybe running the steps is not a good idea."

A TASTE OF HIS OWN MEDICINE

I knew it wasn't his spirit talking; it was his tired body testing me. If I were to agree, that would be the out he needed to say we'll do it next time. I felt Doug needed a little motivation. I reminded him of what he regularly tells Ashley and me, as well as others he works with: "You are committed to what you confess." If you say you'll do something, by golly, he will encourage you to be a person of your word. So I was determined to hold him to his and give him a taste of his own medicine.

I knew this would be a victory for Doug, one we would reflect upon as a milestone in his journey. When we returned to Houston, he was scheduled at MD Anderson for tests and treatment. I didn't want him to regret missing the opportunity to see his vision come to pass.

We arrived at the Parkway Museums District without any problems, found a parking spot, gathered our things in a backpack, and off we went. When Doug saw the Flags of the Nations, he beamed with excitement and was ready to run off without me.

He took a swig of water and put on his do-rag to capture any sweat that would roll down his bald head. I asked if I could follow and capture his run on video using my cell phone. He agreed to slow down for me on occasion, but told me, "I'm on a mission. You can capture me if you can keep up with me." And with that, Doug was off. I hit "play" on the camera app and started running and recording.

The tradition of displaying flags of many countries on the parkway started in 1976 as a part of the United States Bicentennial celebration. There are more than a hundred international flags, representing countries with significant populations in Philadelphia. With a few exceptions, they are hung alphabetically. It is truly a beautiful sight.

INTERCEDING FOR THE NATIONS

Doug ran the trail once and felt so good that he ran it again, interceding for the nations while running. When I caught up to him, we were near the Rocky Statue. People were lined up to take photos. I was still shooting video and asked him what he prayed for. He said, "I prayed for Philadelphia, the City of Brotherly Love, and the headwaters of our nation. I prayed for

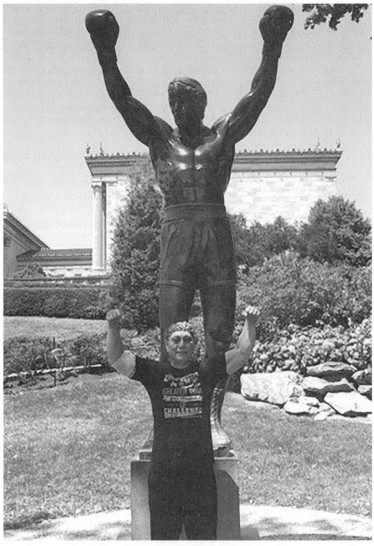

Doug poses at the Rocky Statue. After runing the trail along the Flags of the Nations twice, he also ran up the "Rocky steps" twice.

Houston and the church of America to reach the nations in a tangible way. I prayed as I felt led as I ran past the flags of the numerous nations."

He was sweaty, winded, but full of life. He was the same zealous Doug I knew before cancer. Who he was before the treatments was very much who stood before me—a man who believes that every day is a good day because he serves a great God. The toll cancer had taken on his body wasn't as evident. He had supernatural strength and a desire to win that was greater than his moment of challenge.

We were now at the bottom of the seventy-two steps leading up to the art museum. Looming in front of us was the site of one of the most memorable scenes in *Rocky*.

GOD'S GRACE IS SUFFICIENT

Tourists were everywhere, speaking many languages, and in their midst was Doug. I asked him a question for the video and he said, "I want to be reminded of what it says in 2 Corinthians 12:9: *'My grace is sufficient for you, for My strength is made perfect in weakness.'* Some translations use the word *power* instead of *strength*. I believe the strength and power of God enable us to overcome anything, even in our weak moments. God's grace is sufficient for us. God wants us to all be victorious no matter what we are going through."

I was so moved by what I'd witnessed thus far and thankful that he remained committed to what he confessed. He ran as he said he would. I was about to witness my champion give cancer a good kick in the butt, demonstrating that it won't take away his fight nor his trust in the Lord. I envisioned what was about to happen; Doug at the top of the stairs doing the victory pose. The thought gave me teary eyes.

People all around us were doing the same thing, running up the steps and doing the victory pose at the top. I didn't know their stories or what the run meant to them, but I celebrated with each one who made it, some even shouting and grunting victorious sounds.

Because I couldn't keep up with him on his run, I asked Doug to give me grace. After all, I was trying to capture the

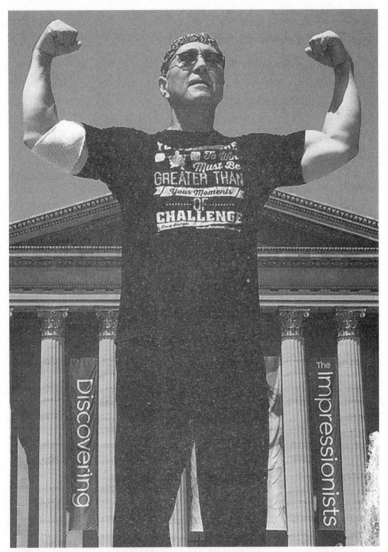

Doug flexes his muscles after running up the steps to the Philadelphia Museum of Art.

moment on video while running up the stairs behind him. Doug gave me a big smile and said, "Ready?"

I hit the record button and chased him. Once again, I lagged behind, but only because it was challenging to keep the camera on him while jogging up the stairs.

There's something about champions and winners that's attractive, especially when they have a humble spirit and have overcome extreme challenges or difficult circumstances. Every generation needs heroes, men and women we can look up to and emulate. Doug reminds us often of the heroic believers in the Bible who obeyed God and accomplished mighty deeds in difficult situations. When we struggle, Doug reminds us, as God's Word does, to consider their faith and imitate their manner of life.

Doug knew people noticed him, watching closely the play-by-play of this journey and how he responded to it. He understood his responsibility, but more than anything, he wanted to please God, not knowing what tomorrow held, but trusting God's control of it. Hebrews 6:12 (NIV) says, "*We do not want you to become lazy, but to imitate those who through faith and patience inherit what has been promised.*" He refused to use cancer as an excuse to become lazy or a reason to stray from his faith. This was not a time to fall back, but to press forward, and, as Hebrews 13:7 says, to imitate the heroes of faith who'd gone before him.

Doug made it to the top, just as he said he would. His smile will forever be engraved in my memory and treasured in my heart. I was still recording as I approached him. He looked at the camera and said, "I believe in God!" He knew where his strength had come from. He was grateful that God allowed him to run the pathway of the Flags of the Nations twice, run up the steps like Rocky did, and do his victory pose. He said, "I've got my victory going on because of Christ Jesus in me. I'm regaining my strength by keeping my vision of hope and keeping my eyes fixed on the brightness of the Son."

ONE MORE TIME!

He was so pumped that when we made it down to the bottom of the steps, he said, "Wait here. I want to run it one more time." This was his well-deserved moment and for me, it was one of the best days ever. Running the *Rocky* steps is a cool thing to do on any given day, but for anyone with a story or a significant meaning behind their run, this becomes truly monumental.

Pastor Rusty Griffin once shared that he no longer looks for medals, but for scars. He said that cancer was a scar and that the scars Jesus has on His body will remain there forever.

Doug and our family would be forever marked by the scar of cancer. Undoubtedly, it deeply marked me, but it wasn't all negative. I am a better person for the experiences I lived. I'm more sensitive to others' needs, seeing beyond what the eye sees, trying to see with my heart, giving grace in greater measure. I am particularly sensitive to anyone who's encountered cancer on any level, whether patient or caregiver, recognizing there is always more than meets the eye.

> IN THE MIDST OF WHATEVER CHAOS SURROUNDS YOU, THERE IS ALWAYS HOPE. DETERMINE TO MAKE TODAY A GOOD DAY. THERE IS NOTHING IMPOSSIBLE FOR GOD.

In the midst of whatever chaos surrounds you, there is always hope. Hug your loved ones, forgive those who come against you, lend someone a helping hand, and don't put off for tomorrow what you can do today, for tomorrow is not promised. Determine to make today a good day. Keep your vision of hope and trust in the Lord for strength. There is nothing impossible for Him.

ANOTHER ROCKY MOMENT

We enjoy watching movies at home more than at the movie theater. We can snuggle, eat lots of popcorn without going broke, and put the movie on pause for restroom breaks. Later in our journey, we decided to watch *Creed*, a sequel to the Rocky movies, for one of our movie nights.

In *Creed*, Sylvester Stallone's character, Rocky, is close to Doug's age. He's a man who is still fit, much like Doug, and a good guy who has been through some things. We hadn't seen the trailer, but took someone's recommendation of it. What they didn't tell us was that Rocky would be diagnosed with Stage 4 non-Hodgkin's lymphoma, the same cancer that Doug was battling.

The moment in the movie when Rocky received the diagnosis, tears streamed down Doug's face. He took some deep breaths, trying to control them, but was unsuccessful. That intensified the tears that flowed uncontrollably from my eyes and down to my neck. I tried to find a way to wipe them without him noticing, but it was obvious. Ashley was in tears too. From that point forward, we were all undone.

I was emotionally involved with the character and found myself recalling specific moments in our own walk. The film has a scene where Donnie, a young boxer, and a frail Rocky run the steps outside the Philadelphia Museum of Art, just like he'd done in prior movies. Doug is very sentimental and tends to shed a few tears during emotional movie scenes. I, on the other hand, try to play the tough cookie, blowing air toward my eyes, quickly wiping away tears, and hoping no one notices that I cried. But this movie choked all of us up. We passed around the tissues during multiple scenes.

Research has proved that it's good to cry and release steam, pressure, and emotions. I agree. When people who are newly dealing with a cancer diagnosis share their hearts with me, many ask how to be strong for their families, I tell them it's okay to cry. Crying is not a sign of weakness or lack of trust in God.

> EVERYONE'S CIRCUMSTANCES ARE DIFFERENT.
> DO WHAT IS BEST FOR YOU AND YOUR FAMILY. WE ARE EACH
> BEAUTIFULLY AND WONDERFULLY MADE, WITH UNIQUE HANDPRINTS
> AND UNIQUE PERSONALITIES.

Everyone's circumstances are different. Write your own story and do what is best for you and your family. There is no rulebook and certainly don't compare yourself to others. We are each beautifully and wonderfully made, with unique handprints and unique personalities.

I have heard it said that tears are liquid prayers. If that is true, let me tell you, I have prayed a lot. Psalm 56:8 (TPT) says, *"You've kept track of all my wandering and my weeping. You've stored my many tears in your bottle—not one will be lost. For they are all recorded in your book of remembrance."*

Watching *Creed* that evening made Doug's run on the pathway of the flags and up the stairs of the museum even more significant. I'm sure I will always cry when I see that scene in any of the *Rocky* movies. It will always be special and will remind me that Doug is a champion who refused to quit, as well as one who practices what he preaches.

CANCER CLAIMS A GENTLE GIANT

We are used to God bringing people into our lives in unexpected ways. My sister, Marisa Scope, had been friends with Greg Bozdech, a coworker, for about nine years. Greg had worked for the city of Pearland, Texas, starting out as a fire investigator and inspector and was eventually promoted to battalion chief fire marshal. He was instrumental in starting the K-9 Accelerant Detection Program and was known all over town as the partner of the first accelerant detection dog, a yellow Labrador retriever named Buddy.

Marisa described Greg as a gentle man who always had a smile on his face, loved his family deeply, and loved serving. He was even-tempered and brought peace to his surroundings.

When Marisa noticed Greg wasn't his joyful self, she asked him if everything was okay. He told her he'd recently been diagnosed with cancer and wanted to be there for his wife and son. Marisa and her coworkers were heartbroken for Greg and his family. They encouraged him as much as they could and kept the family in their prayers. In one of their conversations, Marisa told Greg about Doug's cancer journey, even showing him some of the short videos that Mike May produced and made available on YouTube. Greg was intrigued by our story and asked if she would connect us. He wanted to meet Doug and she couldn't introduce us soon enough.

Doug was at a local coffee shop in Pearland when his phone rang. It was Greg, asking if Doug had any time to meet with him. Doug said, "How about now? I'm in your city and would be happy to meet and pray with you." The two met and felt an instant connection. Greg was greatly admired for his work and Doug considered it an honor to know him. Greg sent us occasional updates and Doug always encouraged him with Scripture. He also called and prayed for Greg as he felt led.

One day, I got a text from Marisa, asking us to pray as Greg was in the hospital. Doug and I were on the road and promised to touch base as soon as we returned to Houston. We decided to stop at the hospital to pray with Greg and his wife. We had just missed her, but he was awake and in good spirits, much like Marisa described him. He was a giant to me, as I am only five-feet-two, yet he had a gentle spirit.

We had communion elements with us and asked if he would like to take communion. His face lit up. Doug led us in prayer, then we celebrated communion together and talked about the future. He reminded us that he wanted to run the *Rocky* steps with Doug someday. His face glowed as he imagined them both doing the victory pose at the top of the steps. Greg also talked about his family and looked forward to all of us meeting someday.

CANCER CLAIMS BOTH PARTNERS

In a tragic coincidence, Buddy died of rapid onset cancer in March 2016. And his partner, Greg, never got to run the *Rocky* steps with Doug. The Lord took him into glory in September 2018. We heard Greg's home-going celebration was beautiful. He was honored with a procession as citizens and public servants lined both sides of the road. Someday, Doug and I will make it back to Philadelphia and run the steps in Greg's honor. He did better than run the steps made famous in a movie. Greg is walking, and maybe even running, on the streets of gold with his heavenly Father, the ultimate victory for those who believe in God.

10

I'M NOT YOUR MOTHER!

I don't remember when in our marriage I began taking my husband's shoes off for him, but it's become a habit in certain situations. Perhaps it started as a way for me to help him relax when I saw him come home from the office, physically drained or emotionally spent. He would sit in the lounge chair in our bedroom to unwind from the busy day and relax after contending with the traffic in a big city. Like many commuters, his drive home could be forty-five minutes to an hour, minimum, on any given day. We didn't have room in our bedroom then for two chairs, so whoever got to the chair first enjoyed it.

At times when he came home not wanting to talk, I took off his shoes, extended the lounge chair, left him a cup of extra hot coffee on the end table next to him, gave him a kiss, dimmed the lights, and left him in peace. Proverbs 21:9 says, *"Better to dwell in a corner of a housetop, than in a house shared with a contentious woman."* I am determined not to be a nagging wife, knowing he would share his day or whatever is heavy on his mind or heart, if and when he's ready.

I've always catered to Doug on his work days, making him that cup of coffee and sitting at his feet. I'm still agile enough to enjoy sitting on the floor while leaning on the chair or our bed. It was an opportunity for me to ask about his day, for him to share whatever was on his heart, and for us to engage in conversations about anything and everything before Ashley joined the party.

Doug often says, "A man who is secure in his identity in Christ is not intimidated by the strengths and gifting of women; rather, he celebrates and cherishes them." In a world so adverse to manhood for the sake of women's "equality," I've heard of women being offended when a man opens the door for them. I'm sure that some women would never consider taking their spouse's shoes off. Doug doesn't expect it, nor demand that I do it. This has nothing to do with equal rights, submission, or any other label. It was, and is, a way for me to spend quality time with my husband as he shares his heart. Why just sit there and listen when I can speed up the process of him relaxing and opening up?

HE RETURNS LOVING GESTURES

In our home, we talk about sowing into our future. Although it started as a way to love on him while spending a vital part of the day together, I have reaped benefits for sowing in love. I get plenty of foot rubs and special treatment from Doug. He takes good care of our family, provides peace in our home, and makes sure I feel valued. Taking off his shoes is simply me being me with the man I'm blessed to love and care for, a way that corresponds to the treatment I receive from him. It's something I don't even think about, just something I do.

There were plenty of hills and valleys throughout our journey. On the day of the first chemotherapy treatment, the abnormal mass in Doug's neck was plain to see. It was the cancer-affected lymph nodes. After each treatment and in subsequent days, we felt the swelling in his neck go down. We assumed and hoped this was a sign that the cancer cells in the lymph nodes throughout his body and his liver were also decreasing.

One day, Doug came home, sat in his chair, and was quiet. He confessed that it had been a physically challenging day, he felt fatigued, then shared a specific concern. His throat bothered him when eating or swallowing. Some of the lymph nodes seemed larger.

I'm sure a tug of war raged between his mind, heart, and emotions. *Was the medicine working? Were all the extra precautions and protocol even making a difference?* With lips closed, he took a deep breath and looked me in the eyes without saying a word. I stood there, trying to figure out what to say. Almost in a whisper, he asked me to stand in front of him and see if I noticed any changes. I wanted to tell him it was just his imagination, that he was tired, and reading something into nothing...but that wasn't the case.

ANOTHER OPPORTUNITY FOR GOD

Unfortunately, I had to agree with him. I saw a bit of new swelling around his neck and chin. I didn't want to discourage Doug, but I couldn't lie. In fact, he says I have the worst poker face ever. So, with that in mind, I told Doug this was just evidence that we were still in an intense battle with more obstacles to overcome.

Doug sat quietly, running his hand up and down his throat, pausing at times to feel the swollen glands, and occasionally taking deep breaths. Then he looked at me and said, "Every obstacle and adversity is an opportunity for God to show Himself greater."

> EVERY OBSTACLE AND ADVERSITY IS AN OPPORTUNITY FOR GOD TO SHOW HIMSELF GREATER. —DOUG

I had not said a word. While he thought, I stood in front of him, interceding in my heart and mind, praying for peace that surpasses understanding, and for healing to manifest in his body.

Doug has an incredible way of bouncing back from gloomy situations. He ponders the negative feelings, considers the evidence, meditates on the Word of God, and then responds according to the promise within him.

Doug often tells us to draw from the deep well within us that never runs dry because it comes from a source that never ceases: the throne room of God. When we intentionally read and study the Bible, we are consuming it. Scriptures can then be brought to recall, especially in times of need. God's Word is life, gives strength, and is hope for the hopeless.

In the end, we chose not to stress or allow our minds to get carried away with negative thoughts. We reminded ourselves of Hebrews 11:1—*"Now faith is the substance of things hoped for, the evidence of things not seen"*—and prayed with confidence, declaring our trust in the Lord.

After dinner, we settled into the family room to watch the news and spend time together. Doug pulled out his calendar and shared his schedule with me. He discussed ministry

assignments already on the calendar and others that were pos-
sibilities. We talked about pacing himself, making sure he had
times of rest.

Something in our conversation struck a nerve. Doug stood
up and said, "If you take the passion of my heart away, which is
to serve the Lord and love people, I might as well die anyway.
The whole purpose of my existence is not about me. It is about
advancing the kingdom of God with the gospel of good news to
see salvation, healing, freedom, and liberation come to others.
So, if you take that calling of God away from me, spreading the
message of the gospel of good news, then I might as well not
even be here. God knows my appointed time and our season."

I just sat and listened. I understood where he was coming
from and knew this to be true. Hard as it was, I would have to
trust that Doug knew his limits, when he needed to slow down,
and when he could push the envelope.

One week, I'd noticed that Doug was full of energy while
at the pulpit. But after he finished, his voice was hoarse and his
body a bit worn out. I'd read of other ministers with similar
experiences. Some had been brought to the pulpit in a wheelchair, stood and preached a fiery sermon, and when done, were
too weak to walk, once again needing the wheelchair. With that
in mind, I wasn't too concerned. I figured it would be part of
Doug's story, another example of someone who preached the
gospel, seemingly full of life, but when it was over, felt weak and
depleted.

This time, however, someone at the host church noticed his
faded voice as we were leaving church and asked me if he was
okay. They had watched Doug's energy level drop after he finished and were blown away by what God had done in the service. I told them Doug had made it clear to me, and those near

to him, that if sharing the love of the Lord was taken from him, it would not be good for his spirit. He was doing what he loved to do, but he needed a bit more rest at the end of the day. The pastor understood that Doug was operating in an anointing of God for the assignment before him and was grateful to have had him minister.

During this season, Doug continued to write articles and blogs. Various online magazines and a television network asked for permission to repost or publish his articles through which we continued to declare God's goodness. We determined to let His light shine in and through us in every way possible. Serving God was Doug's plumb line of stability. His foundations were unshakable because God is of the unshakable kingdom.

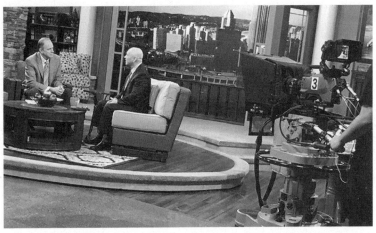

Tom Hollis of Cornerstone TV interviews Doug on the program Real Life.

When talking about the diagnosis and treatments, Doug explained that he could not put his hope in medical professionals, whom he trusted, respected, and honored. His hope remained in the Lord. He would receive and appreciate the medical care, but God alone had the ultimate say in this journey.

Doug knew his physical ability came from the strength of his spiritual relationship with God. The commitment Doug made to read Scripture, pray, and spend significant time with the Lord helped his mind to not become distracted or disillusioned. It kept his focus and his faith on the One who always keeps His promises. That was a vital part of his strategy.

TASTY TREATS STILL BANISHED

I didn't keep what most folks call junk food or tasty treats in the house once we determined to make the dietary changes we felt necessary to help Doug beat this disease. For a long time, desserts of any kind were neither purchased nor made at the home. I imagine many are feeling sorry for Doug but especially for Ashley. *What kid doesn't like cookies, ice cream, or cake after dinner?* Doug shared my restrictions with the world as he humorously posted them on social media.

Some people made him dessert and took it to the office. A few friends even made what they called healthy delicacies and found a way to deliver them to wherever he was preaching. I eventually experimented with baking healthy desserts, but I never mastered the art of making them delicious, so I just gave up. I'm still a work-in-progress in the kitchen.

I didn't eat or drink things that weren't good for Doug when he was home. I tried to avoid them altogether, but was guilty of enjoying certain foods when he wasn't home or we were apart. The joke around the house was, "Do as I say, not as I do." I still bought potato chips on occasion to enjoy with a sandwich, and my mom enjoyed having her own treats.

Mom's doctor had told us that her cholesterol and sugar levels were marginally high, but nothing to worry about if she exercised self-control and continued her normal diet. At her age, the doctor said Mom could enjoy chocolate ice cream if she wanted. Then she looked at Mom and said, "Just don't eat it every day." With that in mind, Mom put things on my grocery list that made her taste buds happy, but were on my "absolutely no way" list for Doug. I tried to hide them, but Doug had a way of finding them and occasionally enjoying them.

One evening, I walked to where Doug sat comfortably in his chair and took my favorite spot at his feet. I reminded him that he shouldn't be breaking the at-home protocol. I asked him to stop surreptitiously eating the chips and any other foods that weren't part of the winning strategy.

CHIPS NOT PART OF CANCER PROTOCOL

It's not that he was doing it behind my back. Doug just enjoyed them when I wasn't around to tell him to put them down. Maybe he thought I wouldn't mind, or maybe he wanted to enjoy things his taste buds had previously savored. After all, he drank and ate everything I put before him. Maybe he felt he deserved a treat every now and then.

It was apparently the wrong day and wrong time to ask him to give up the treats because the answer I got back was not what I expected. Doug looked at me with frustration and spoke with annoyance. "Stop being my mother. You're not my mother!"

I felt crushed and wanted to cry, but didn't want him to see how deeply those words had wounded me. We sat in silence. Our eyes locked for a moment, communicating without words. He leaned back in his chair. I blinked and let my head drop, trying to find the words to change the atmosphere.

In a soft voice, I apologized for being so strict. I tried to explain, in as few words as possible, that I was just looking out for him. After all, what *could* I say to someone I'd promised to eat and drink everything he would, then at the first try failed miserably? Perhaps I was like a military drill sergeant, wanting more than anything to see my soldier make it through boot camp.

Doug reminded me he was a grown man and didn't need me telling him what to do. I wasn't in his shoes, drinking and eating all the unpleasant protocols that he endured. I wasn't being humbled by needing help wrapping the PICC line before every bath. I wasn't dependent on my spouse to flush that PICC line daily and change the medical dressing every week. He was tired, displeased, frustrated, irritated, and on that day, he'd had enough and told me just how he felt.

I excused myself and went to one of the bathrooms. A hand towel muffled my cries and tissues wiped the steady tears. I leaned my back against the wall and slid down until I was squatting on the floor, my elbows on my knees and my hands covering my face. I was a tired, hurt, and emotional mess.

PULLED IN ALL DIRECTIONS

During this season, I'd become an in-home and traveling nurse and head dietician. Making meals for the family was more time consuming than before as I learned how to cook in a completely different manner. I paid more attention to the ingredients of every prepared meal and bought as much organic food as possible. I spent twice as much time at the grocery store, no longer grabbing items I was used to getting, but checking the ingredients of each item. It was a tedious but necessary chore.

At home, I constantly wiped everything, especially door handles and commonly touched areas, to kill any germs that could be passed on to Doug. I was still wife, mother, and caregiver for my mother, a homeschooling mom, ministry leader, friend, chauffeur, and more.

Since Doug wasn't slowing down much, this meant the same for me. I woke up before anyone else, got a head start on the day, and enjoyed quiet time with the Lord—and usually ended my days well after midnight.

Most days were good, but some were wearing. In addition to Doug's cancer, Ashley dealt with challenges as well. She needed more of my time when I felt like I had less. We had also committed time for ministering to many others who were walking through cancer journeys or other challenges. While witnessing some of what they were going through took a toll on me, it also drove me to go before the altar of God in prayer and intercession.

FINANCIAL CHALLENGES, TOO

Beyond the physical exhaustion, there was the emotional rollercoaster and financial challenges to maneuver. One time, I received a call from the hospital, informing me that we owed a large sum of money. This was the first time I'd heard about it. I told them we couldn't come up with the full amount at once, but were willing to make payments. The bottom line was if we didn't pay it all, we couldn't continue with the treatments. My heart shattered at that moment. We couldn't stop the chemotherapy. Once treatment starts, you may feel better, but it must be completed to be fully effective.

I hung up, rested my head on my arms, and cried out to God. *How could this be possible?* I asked Him to intervene and make a miracle happen. I stayed at my desk, put on worship music, called a friend to share the news, and had her agree with me in prayer for a miracle. She asked if I'd shared this with Doug yet. I hadn't—and had no intention of adding this stress to his plate unless we didn't witness a miracle. Then, he would have to know since his chemotherapy would be interrupted. That alone was a scary thought.

Doug often says, "Out of some of our most challenging and difficult circumstances, out of our moments of pain, God can bring forth some of our greatest testimonies." I had no choice but to believe and pray for the financial miracle and a great testimony.

After a healthy time of crying and interceding, I got it together and called our insurance company regarding the issue. They were concerned for us and said they would make a call on our behalf. Our insurance company is actually a bill-sharing ministry called Medi-Share. Their representatives never fail to ask how they can pray for me or my family at the end of every call. It's been a significant blessing for me. By the time the call ended, I had peace again and decided to see this as a curve ball that God would teach me how to hit.

The miracle happened. Within a short span of time, I received a call, telling me that all was resolved. We could proceed with the treatments scheduled on the following day. My tears of joy and gratitude to the Lord could have filled a cup or two. I went from mourning to gladness, from sorrow to joy, from feeling beaten down and destroyed to flying on wings like an eagle and regaining strength as I soared toward the brightness of the Son.

We'd been dealt a devastating blow, but the love, power, and armor of God changed what was meant to harm us and turned it into good. This was one of those moments when I could get off the emotional rollercoaster I'd been on for the last few hours and say, as Doug says, "Today is a good day because we serve a great God."

TRYING TO EMULATE THE VIRTUOUS WIFE

Some things, like this incident, I never shared with Doug—not because I wanted to keep him in the dark, but because he didn't need the additional worry. I wanted to demonstrate and prove that he had an able and willing wife and didn't need to know the extent of the load I carried beyond what he witnessed.

I try to be like "The Virtuous Wife" in Proverbs 31:10–31, about whom it's said:

> *Who can find a virtuous wife? For her worth is far above rubies. The heart of her husband safely trusts her; so he will have no lack of gain. She does him good and not evil all the days of her life.... She girds herself with strength, and strengthens her arms.... She extends her hand to the poor, yes, she reaches out her hands to the needy.... Her husband is known in the gates, when he sits among the elders of the land.... Strength and honor are her clothing; she shall rejoice in time to come. She opens her mouth with wisdom, and on her tongue is the law of kindness. She watches over the ways of her household, and does not eat the bread of idleness. Her children rise up and call her blessed; her husband also, and he praises her: "Many daughters have done well, but you excel them all." Charm is deceitful and beauty is passing, but a woman who fears the LORD, she shall be praised. Give her of the fruit of her hands, and let her own works praise her in the gates.*

It's not that those who strive to be Proverbs 31 women think that we're anything special. We just know that the Lord is the source of our strength. We aren't superheroes, although our kids may sometimes think we are. We fail, sometimes miserably, but don't give up. We rest in the Lord, worshipping and washing our minds with His Word. Sometimes, we get new insights on how to overcome situations; sometimes, we receive silence and are stretched in our level of trust.

Trying to be this warrior princess at all stages in life is simply part of our calling as wives, mothers, grandmothers, friends, businesswomen, and so much more. If I can be a peacemaker in my home and community, serve and love my family, and participate in their joy as they live, serve, and mature in God, then these are the greatest gifts I can receive.

All things considered, I was never trying to be Doug's mother. That thought never crossed my mind. I only tried to be his loving wife, fighting for his life to the best of my ability. I fought with prayer, the biggest gift I could give him. I prayed and spoke Scripture and life over him every chance I got. I made a covenant with him on our wedding day to love him in sickness and in health, till death do us part. I was only keeping my promise to love him through it all, even on his crabby and cranky days. And he had a few.

Doug was never mean to me, just curt at times. I know I got on his nerves. After all, I was the one who made sure he ate or drank the nasty stuff. I was the one who took away the simple things he enjoyed, like coffee. I caught him drinking it on occasion and took it away after he'd only had a few sips. His diet was always on my mind. We did our best to eliminate sugar because cancer cells feed on it. I also learned that cancer cells will use protein and fat for fuel in the absence of sugar, so I was always trying to avoid the things that could feed these terrible invasive cells.

So, yes, I totally got the mother thing, but I was determined to see this through by ensuring Doug had every possible fighting chance to win this battle. Besides, I wanted him to co-author chapters in our love story for many decades to come.

I was simply his loving wife who refused to give up and wanted him to live. I would stand for whatever he wanted me to stand for and I would hold on to the promises of the Lord no matter what we were going through. We committed to doing this together and were determined to come out of it with a testimony.

I wasn't trying to be Doug's mother. I was trying to keep the gift of my husband.

11

SOWING AND REAPING

The day after coming home from Philadelphia, Doug was scheduled for a PET scan and blood work. The scan was required halfway through the treatment plan. About a week prior to that, Ashley had a dream that Daddy was healed and had a full head of hair again. I could totally embrace that and it was something I looked forward to by faith. A number of friends thought he looked good bald. But I loved his hair and longed to have it back, especially because it would be a sign of his healing.

During that week, I also received a call from Susie Wolf, who dreamt that Doug was writing to thank everyone for all the love and prayers shown to us as we travelled the cancer journey. In the letter, Doug was sharing the news that God was bigger than the cancer that attacked his body. The Big C, Christ Jesus, took out the little c, cancer.

These dreams were encouraging and affirmed that we focus on our destination, not what we were going through. They gave us hope, but we still lived each day knowing we were in a battle and could not let our guard down in any way.

Doug had a full schedule of meetings and missed a call from the hospital. Later in the day, they called again. The hospital was intent on reaching him, making multiple calls to confirm he would be at the scheduled appointment with Dr. Jason Westin. We hadn't missed any appointments and never received reminder calls. We only ever got emails and constantly checked our patient portal to make sure all was in order. Doug found it odd and prayed that the medical team wouldn't have any concerns. We believed for the best, but wondered about the phone calls. We had to take control of our imaginations. Each of us encouraged the other over the next twenty hours.

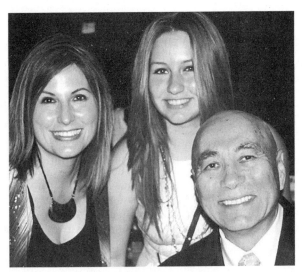

Lisa, Ashley, and Doug Stringer

ASHLEY KNOWS DADDY WILL BE HEALED

Morning came soon enough and with it lots of anticipation. Doug and I spent quality time with the Lord and kept an attitude of gratitude. Ashley and I worshipped in the kitchen as she helped me prepare the not-so-tasty things that Doug needed for breakfast. Ashley bombarded me with a healthy dose of positive reminders that Daddy was healed. "It's just a matter of time," she said, "before we will all see it."

The four of us gathered in the kitchen, held hands, and prayed before Doug and I left for the medical center.

As we waited for the doctor and his team, Doug and I prayed for the many patients who were going through trials at the hospital. We prayed for the medical staff, the families of those in treatment, their financial needs, and so much more. We also gave thanks to God in advance for the complete healing Doug would experience.

"THERE IS NO EVIDENCE OF DISEASE"

Dr. Westin entered the room, took his seat, and didn't waste any time sharing the results. He hung the two scans next to each other. He pointed to the first one, which showed Doug's body riddled with disease. Most of the organs were lit up with evidence of cancer. Then he pointed at the next one and simply said, "There is no evidence of disease."

Talk about a *big* sigh of relief and tears of joy! Doug and I were holding hands. He gave me a squeeze of affirmation and wiped away his tears of gratitude. Dr. Westin was always kind, concerned, and generous with his time when answering our questions. I would recommend him to anyone. But he always had a stoic look and kept conversations to the matters at hand.

This was the first time, out of all of our prior meetings, that I saw a peaceful smile on the doctor's face.

Doug and I knew not all of his patients survived. It must be easier to not get too attached to anyone. I can't imagine the heartbreak doctors must feel when they lose a patient, especially someone they've treated for a long time. Doctors spend hours researching, studying, and consulting others, trying to find a cure for the specific cancer in which they specialize. They invest time helping those in need and answering emergency calls that take them away from their own families. Being an oncologist must involve an emotional cost.

At one of our first meetings, Doug was on the exam table and Dr. Westin was preparing to feel the lymph nodes in Doug's throat and body. I sat in the corner a few feet away. Doug, trying to lighten the mood, told the doctor that I eliminated all sugar from his diet and wouldn't let him have dessert. With a bit of a laugh but a serious tone, Doug said, "Dr. Westin, would you please tell my wife that it's okay for me to have a dessert? A slice of cheesecake would be great, or a piece of apple pie."

I couldn't believe Doug had just called me out like that in front of the doctor! But even more surprising was the doctor's reply. He suggested I let Doug enjoy whatever he wanted to enjoy. I think it took Doug by surprise, too, but he loved every word affirming his request for dessert. He said, "See, honey? Doctor's orders. I'm absolutely going to enjoy it now."

I was not a happy camper on the inside and shocked at his response. All I could think of later was that perhaps they didn't think Doug would make it and the least I could do was let him enjoy whatever he wanted. Or maybe they knew that after chemo started, his taste buds wouldn't desire the same things and he might be too sick to enjoy food. I never asked the doctor why he gave that answer and it really doesn't matter anymore. No matter what he said, I still wouldn't approve of sugary desserts and Doug could do whatever he chose, even if I didn't agree.

...BUT CHEMO MUST CONTINUE

Only halfway through treatments and God showed us again He was and is more than able. I'll never forget Doug's joy and next question. "Does this mean no more chemo?" Dr. Westin said it didn't work that way. It would be nice, but he had to complete the chemotherapy—every last bit of it. A few stray cancer cells might be hiding that weren't detected by the test, he explained. We needed to ensure they were all dead and gone.

Doug responded with his usual word when he doesn't like an outcome: "Bummer." But he wasn't complaining. He knew who had gone before him and who would continue to make a way.

Dr. Westin ordered Doug's next chemo treatment for the next day. Before leaving the examine room, we thanked him again and also thanked God for His wisdom and intervention thus far. We walked out of the room and tried to contain our emotions. No matter what floor we were on or what hallway we walked down, we found people who looked like they were in a battle for their lives—because they were.

We waited until we were far from the busyness of the hospital. In fact, we waited until we neared the exit of the parking garage before we texted the joyous and miraculous news to a few people. Through social media and emails, we shared the news that the scan done after three chemo treatments showed no evidence of cancer. With grateful hearts, we thanked all those who'd covered us in prayer, helped with our financial needs, provided meals, and simply loved us during this season.

Later that day, I wrote in a post:

We rejoice over what only the Lord could have done; He has proven that He is *bigger* than any diagnosis and any weapon formed against His children. We are without words, and full of tears of joy and emotions that cannot be described accurately. To God be the glory! Jesus, You did it! Through it all, we kept Hebrews 12:2 in mind; we did not lose our vision of hope, and we kept our eyes on the author and finisher of our faith.

We couldn't stop saying thank you to the many who kept us encouraged. While overwhelmed with joy, we fully recognized that the battle was not over. Ecclesiastes 3:1–8 says there is a season for everything.

PRESSING FORWARD ON ALL FRONTS

Doug never received this diagnosis as his personally, but as a prophetic drama of the spiritual dynamic of our nation. After more tears of joy, he reminded me that this was not a time to let our guard down, slow down, or cease interceding and praying for our nation. Specifically for us, though the PET scan showed no evidence of disease, this was not a time to let up. So we determined to press forward in communion and prayer on all fronts.

Doug is a man who will always direct you to truth. He often makes statements that cause me to contemplate what I just heard and how it applies to my life. He constantly reminds us to filter what we hear and believe through the Word of God. One of my favorite phrases is, "Perception isn't always the truth, but it is to the one who perceives it." Turn on the news or pay closer attention to conversations you have with people. Take into consideration the facts that you know and you'll find that statement to be true.

With close to four decades in ministry, Doug has experienced and witnessed miracles and breakthroughs. He's survived guns being thrust in his face and has been punched and harassed. I never tire of hearing Doug's stories, especially when there's someone else with us who experienced it with him or was a witness to it. Dual perspectives often bring more color and life to the story. I still get teary when he shares testimonies of people who lived on the streets in hopeless situations. They accepted the kindness of a stranger who did nothing more than demonstrate the love of Christ. Many found healing and their lives were transformed. Relationships that seemed destroyed were restored.

Second Corinthians 5:17 says, "*Therefore, if anyone is in Christ, he is a new creation; old things have passed away; behold, all things have become new.*" I know of young women who previously had been involved in prostitution who today are healthy, educated, working women and mothers. They were made new and are making a difference in society and the kingdom of God.

In December 1996, Doug was led to host a corporate time of fasting, prayer, and worship known as Houston's Prayer Mountain. He rented an amphitheater on the only spot in Houston where there was a small hill, where you can sit on the lawn and enjoy concerts. For those unfamiliar with the Houston landscape, the city is relatively flat and barely above sea level. For forty days, people gathered for services lasting five to six hours. Pastors and believers alike were touched throughout the greater Houston area. God subsequently moved mightily and reached nations all over the globe.

I've been fortunate to travel with Doug to six continents and over thirty-four nations, meeting people who shared how significant that prayer gathering was for them or someone they knew. I've seen the tears of joy and heard the laughter when they reminisce about the pivotal experience that transformed them into who they are today.

AN AMAZING HARVEST REAPED

At that prayer meeting in Houston, Doug sowed the seed that would reap an unimaginable harvest during our season of cancer nearly nineteen years later. It was one that only God could have brought forth and made plentiful. There's no way this story could have been any better than the way the Lord allowed the miracle to take place and be known. It is truly a testimony to the goodness and grace of God, who is omniscient and omnipotent.

On September 10, 2015, Doug and I were in Dallas for a fundraising banquet for United Cry/DC16 to protect life, promote the role of pastors in America, and pray for revival and awakening. Doug served on the steering committee and was honored to be one of the speakers. As always, I felt blessed to hear Doug and the others minister to and encourage us. But this evening and this message were extra special. My warrior soared on his eagle's wings as God had His way in Doug's life and ministry. We gave the Lord all the glory due His name.

As Doug closed out his segment, noticeably full of energy and his bald head shining, he told a little bit about his cancer journey and the results of the latest PET scan. The audience applauded, but the speech wasn't about Doug. It was about God's faithfulness, about all of us as intercessors being unshaken in our faith and trust in God.

Jack Hayford has said, "Faith must have a resting place. When deep sufferings threaten the foundations of faith, we must be firmly rooted in His truths." Faith had a resting place in Doug's heart and it was evident. The testimony encouraged those in attendance to not lose hope, remain steadfast in God's Word, and be people of prayer accompanied by the faith that moves mountains.

MEETING A MIGHTY WARRIOR

One of Doug's greatest passions is sowing into the next generations. He gives freely to those who hunger for truth and righteousness and will pay it forward. Doug will be the first to tell you, "Silver and gold I have none, but what I have I will share, including my relational equity." The Bible says, *"Iron sharpens iron"* (Proverbs 27:17) and Doug also gleans from the young visionaries and kingdom warriors, usually leaving these encounters feeling motivated, hopeful, and inspired.

At the close of the banquet, we met a young man who had been fasting and praying for Doug. It turned out that the two of them had actually met before. Derek Sewell was a handsome young man with a long, bushy beard and golden hair that was tied in a bun near his neck. Dressed in a suit, he towered over Doug. Derek told us that in 2005, when he was just eighteen, he lost his father to esophageal cancer. As he shared his heart, I teared up with gratitude for the mighty warrior before me and what God had done through him, without my knowing.

The first time Derek heard Doug speak, he was sitting across the room from him in a steering committee meeting. Doug had said, "At this national prayer gathering, we don't need preachers pontificating or politicians giving speeches. America is desperate and we need the presence of God." That sparked a fire in Derek and the hope that an older generation genuinely cared about the presence of God in his generation. Derek said he was thankful for all of the preachers in the community and nation, but to hear Doug say that God showing up mattered more than anything hit home.

Derek recounted how he and two other young men felt after being with Doug one afternoon at a coffee shop. "We left that meeting just blown away," he said. "It was like hanging out with your dad. I don't have a dad, so just to see this guy with such a genuine heart and love for God and love for people spoke volumes."

> **HOPELESSNESS CAN BE A CONTINUOUS BATTLE FOR CHILDREN AND YOUTH WHO MISS OUT ON A FATHER'S PRESENCE, LOVE, AFFIRMATION, ACCEPTANCE, AND APPROVAL.**

Sometime after that meeting, Derek heard about Doug's cancer and he knew too many national prayer leaders had died from cancer. "I'm sick of it, so tired of it, Lord," he said. "We don't need to lose another one." After serving in young adult and youth ministry for years, Derek knew the problems created when families lacked fathers. Hopelessness can be a continuous battle for children and youth who miss out on a father's presence, love, affirmation, acceptance, and approval.

HEARING FROM GOD

Derek later had a dream where he heard the voice of the Lord. He said he doesn't have prophetic dreams often, but this one really shook him. He said God told him, "Doug Stringer is a father to this generation and if you fast and pray and intercede for his healing, you'll be praying and interceding for the fathers in America."

Derek said he got chills just recalling the dream. He asked the Lord, "How can I fast and pray? Is this like a three-day fast? A twenty-one-day fast? Lord, what are you wanting? Holy Spirit, show me." He was reminded that Jesus said, *"By this everyone will know that you are my disciples, if you love one another"* (John

13:35 NIV). He determined to give all that he had and started a forty-day fast. He wanted Doug to know he was fully loved.

We were overwhelmed and humbled that this young man, who had been led into a spiritual Nazarene consecration to the Lord, would make such a sacrifice to agree for Doug's healing and calling. Derek also told us that he'd recently had a dream that Doug was healed.

THE HARVEST COMES FULL CIRCLE

Amazingly, Derek's wife, Melissa, then his fiancée, decided to encourage, support, and partner with him by joining his fast for Doug's healing. He had only told her about the fast so she wouldn't question his crazy new eating habits. It meant a lot to Derek when she decided to fast with him because he noticed how Doug and I ministered together.

In one of Melissa's conversations with her parents, she mentioned that she and Derek were fasting for Doug—and to her surprise, they knew Doug. They are missionary pastors in Mexico City and have served there for over thirty years. They visited Houston in December 1996, heard about the forty-day fasting and prayer gathering, and decided to attend.

During those prayer gatherings, Doug never took an offering for the ministry. Some people chose to sow anyway and would leave jewelry at the altar. But Doug let those in attendance know that if they needed resources, they could take from whatever was offered, cashing it in to meet their needs or doing with it whatever they felt led to do. It was between them and God.

Melissa's parents gave whatever they had to the people they served in Mexico City. They loved what they were called to do and lived a sacrificial lifestyle, giving their all to the ministry.

When you serve the less fortunate, you don't worry about fine jewelry or name brands. Your focus is loving people in truth and being a visible expression of His love. But Melissa's mom had a mother's heart and she prayed the Lord would provide her with some pretty jewelry that she could pass down to her daughters.

Doug had no idea of the desires of this mother's heart, but God did. Melissa's parents had gone to the Houston Prayer Mountain gatherings in 1996 and never imagined they would end up with an heirloom for their beautiful daughter. Decades later, at her wedding, they presented it to her. It didn't have great financial value, but because it was an answer to prayer, it was a gift from God Himself. Doug's obedience to not sell the jewelry for funds to meet the needs of the ministry, but to pay it forward led to this legacy.

At the United Cry/DC16 fundraising banquet in 2015, Derek heard for the first time that Doug's cancer was in remission. His fast had ended the day before.

Derek's forty-day fasting assignment on Prayer Mountain Dallas was part of a legacy that began in 1996 during a fasting call at Houston's Prayer Mountain nearly twenty years earlier. Doug sowed a gift of jewelry to some missionaries desiring an heirloom for their daughter, who would eventually become Derek's bride. He fasted and prayed for the man who sowed the bracelet worn by Melissa, his beautiful bride, on their wedding day.

Writing about the full-circle harvest later, Derek wrote:

> Lisa started weeping and said, "Thank you so much for praying." I saw that genuineness. It was my first time ever meeting her and seeing how she genuinely thanked me was crazy. All I did was pray. But I know there was a sacrifice to it, seeing her heart and how real

and authentic she was. How much she loves her husband. She told us how Doug prays on his knees daily for my generation. For someone to say that, says a lot, but for his own wife to give testimony about him— that's amazing. You don't hear things like that. To hear a couple laying down their lives for a generation, that's nuts. And that's what we need more of. We need more fathers and mothers to show a generation that somebody does care.

God took my little seed of faith, that I was sowing with only my fiancée's knowledge and I was given the privilege of seeing Doug healed. Every time I think about it, I say, "God, thank you! That's a father we haven't lost!" Think about all the sons and all the daughters who are going to come as a result of this man's life. So perhaps you can see that this tapestry was so much bigger than I could have ever imagined it to be.

My wife and I are thankful. I know I don't have a dad but God has shown me through this whole process that I am not fatherless. He redeems our lives and our stories. I am so thankful that God has woven the lives of the Stringers, my family, and extended family together for an amazing story. You can't make this kind of stuff up. I have been impacted for the rest of my life. I can't deny it. That would be insane. That would be like someone trying to tell me that gravity isn't real. God is real and He loves people and He gave His Son who died on the cross for us and rose again. He did it all for us. The gospel is real and I'll spend the rest of my life preaching this. I'm just thankful for the journey. I am thankful for Doug, I am thankful for Lisa.

ANSWERING A NUDGE FROM GOD

The person who gave that bracelet may never know of the joy they brought a sacrificial, loving, and generous mom as she blessed her daughter with a tender gift on her wedding day. When God nudges you to give, just do it. Remember, obedience is the highest form of worship.

Doug often says, "Prayer is so much more than handing a list of requests to God. If you want earth-shaking results, you will be required to travail until heaven's plan becomes a reality on earth."

Derek and Melissa, thank you for travailing. To the many who went to their knees on our behalf and travailed with us, thank you. I'm sure there are many war room champions who partnered in prayer with us who I will never know about on this side of heaven. Just know that we thank you and recognize that you, too, were a vital part of our victory through Christ Jesus.

> NO MATTER WHAT UNEXPECTED DETOURS YOU ENCOUNTER, GOD WANTS US TO KEEP OUR FOCUS ON WHERE WE'RE GOING, NOT WHAT WE ARE GOING THROUGH.

For the Sewells and the Stringers, God had already established His purposes over twenty years ago. Never take for granted what you go through, good or bad. Allow it to be turned for the good because God has a greater story that comes out of your place of need. No matter what unexpected detours you encounter, God wants us to keep our focus on where we're going, not what we are going through.

12

JOURNEY ON

Life continued after receiving the news that the chemotherapy was working. We carried on with our workload, as well as the scheduled treatments. Doug and the team were in the middle of organizing two more national prayer gatherings: one in North Carolina and the other in Orlando, Florida.

On one of our scheduled travel days, we were stuck at the airport for about fourteen hours. Our original flight had been delayed numerous times and eventually canceled. Just before boarding our newly scheduled flight, the captain decided that the plane needed two tires changed, which caused more delay. We made it to Raleigh around 2 a.m., checked into a room for an hour and a half, and then headed back to the airport for our connecting flight to the original destination.

We were sleepless in North Carolina, yet full of expectation. Excitement filled the air. Pastors of many denominations, races, and all generations made a commitment to join the solemn assembly scheduled for September 26.

After the meetings, I managed to squeeze in a thirty-minute nap before our three-and-a-half-hour road trip to South Carolina. We laughed as we reflected on the challenges of the last thirty-six hours. While at the airport on our return flight, Doug's watch broke as he took it off to go through security check. To top it off, so did his luggage. We were so tired, we couldn't help but laugh at all that happened to us. It was unreal. We chose to have a merry heart with every new challenge. Not to say there wasn't evidence of us being tired. We certainly looked a little worn and with every step, we moved slower. Nonetheless, we pressed in. God is faithful and we were grateful for the opportunity to partner with so many to do kingdom business.

On one of the treatment days, we were blessed to visit with friends and a fellow patient who drove in for his follow-up testing. He received a good report. Many of the patients we knew were from out of town and booked themselves at one of the extended stay motels near the medical center during their outpatient treatment days. The waiting areas, atriums, and cafes were often our gathering places for those we knew who were also undergoing treatment or testing on the same days we were.

Mike May called the places we settled in "the war rooms." When I looked through photographs taken during the journey, there were numerous videos and pictures of us holding hands with our heads bowed in a posture of prayer. A powerful sight for me is to see patients with their white identification bracelets embracing other patients and praying for one another. It's a compelling visual and one that must touch the heart of God.

By the time round five of chemo was almost over, I was physically and emotionally worn out. I knew that a thankful heart was a key to victory and would energize me, as I had to drive us home. From the second chemo on, Ashley brought her guitar to every treatment. She led us in worship not only before the infusions, but as she felt led throughout the day and as the PICC line was disconnected from the medications.

In the room that evening, we praised God and declared our trust in Him for health and strength to continue a full week of ministry. We thanked God for all the prayers we knew were said on our behalf, thanked Him for the continuous love and support we received, and declared that with God, all things were possible. We prayed for the patients in the rooms next to us. Seeing those who were alone, without family or friends, left a heavy burden on my heart.

We were finally released from our assigned room for the day. It had been saturated with prayer and we believed that the next patient would feel God's presence in it. Room 54 was a war room that day and God had His way in it!

THIRTY PILLS COST $1,000

One of the miracles we experienced was Doug's lack of side effects from the chemotherapy. During his first infusion, I was handed a prescription for nausea medication and told to hurry to the pharmacy as they closed in fifteen minutes. This would be nearly impossible since the pharmacy was in another building.

I hustled to the elevator and arrived at the floor that connected the buildings with a skywalk. The extended golf carts that transport patients, family, and staff were full. I had no choice but to run. I'm not a runner, but made it to the pharmacy with two minutes to spare. I turned in the prescription, waited with many others, and tried to act normal. I was breathing hard and had worked up a sweat.

Soon, I saw Doug's name on the "ready" board and approached the counter. The cashier said, "That will be a thousand dollars."

I was suddenly out of breath again. "Excuse me?" I said, certain I'd misunderstood.

He said, "That will be a thousand dollars. Will you be paying with a credit card?"

I asked about discount cards and more, only to find out there were no discounts...and we didn't have prescription coverage. I looked at the dosage and realized this would cost a thousand dollars a month for the next six months. I needed to figure out what to do. I decided to charge this first month's supply, but what about the subsequent months? I would have to trust God to provide.

Miracles come in surprising ways. Doug chose to not take the medicine unless absolutely necessary. The directions recommended it be taken daily to prevent the nausea, but Doug rarely needed it. He felt nauseous at times, but in his mind, not enough to merit taking the medication. Instead, God provided the healing that became part of the financial testimony of His provision.

By His grace, Doug helped facilitate the Response North Carolina on September 26, 2015, in Charlotte. The posture of humble prayer, repentance, and recognition of the Lord's holiness was powerful. The war room prayers resulted in a shift during the preparation for the gatherings and at the event. Unity in our diversity happened because of our common denominator, Jesus. We were privileged to serve in these grassroots efforts, meeting with co-laborers and believers from all over our nation. Above all, we acknowledged God's sovereignty as we gathered to intercede on behalf of our nation and the nations of the world.

We knew God had us right where He wanted us. In the midst of our challenges, He gave us hope and strength to persevere. Our focus now turned to preparing for the Response in Florida on October 24.

It was now September 29, the day of our last chemo infusion. Pastors Steve and Becky Riggle blessed us with their presence and support and led us in communion before the treatment began. They've been a great example of perseverance through trials and adversities. While ministering in a prison in the Philippines years ago, they were held captive and survived being shot and stabbed numerous times.

Once settled, we wasted no time getting our pretreatment protocol started. As I distributed the communion elements, Ashley took out her guitar. We never directed her selection. The songs Ashely chose were always fitting. When she began to sing "What I Know," a song by Tricia Brock, tears of gratitude flowed down my face. The powerful lyrics expressed what many in the hospital probably felt. Just as the song says, "And if it doesn't turn out like I think it should/It doesn't change the fact You're always good."

NO MATTER WHAT, GOD IS ALWAYS GOOD

No matter how you feel, God is real and always good. Those words resonated throughout our journey—on our bad days, our good days, and our better good days. God is real and will forever be real to us.

Pastor Steve had been teaching on the tangible power of God and suggested Doug share that evening at the midweek prayer service. At first, Doug thought Steve was joking. After all, Doug was hooked up to chemo and the negative side effects can be gruesome.

But the invitation was real and Doug accepted it. What better way to thank the Lord for His great grace, strength, and power than to minister in His might that evening? When the session ended, Doug was not just disconnected from the medications, but the PICC line was also removed! He could get back to some semblance of normality, although to his credit, he maintained normality the best he could the entire time.

In another act of faith, we left MD Anderson and drove to Grace Woodlands, making it just in time for service. Doug taught on the power of God out of Philippians 3:10, Exodus 33, and John 13:7 where Jesus said, *"You do not understand now what I am doing, but you will understand later"* (GNT).

> ## GOD GIVES US HIS GRACE THROUGH ALL CIRCUMSTANCES AND TURNS THEM INTO TESTIMONIES OF THE LORD.

It's true that God gives us His grace through all circumstances and turns them into testimonies of the Lord. Only God could sustain a man who leaves his hospital bed to share His goodness immediately after finishing the last of six chemo treatments. As we pulled away from the hospital, a rainbow crossed the sky. It was a perfect reminder of His promises to us.

John 11:40 (NIV) says, *"Then Jesus said, 'Did I not tell you that if you believe, you will see the glory of God?'"* Without a doubt, we experienced His grace, peace, provision, and abounding love. Our desire now was that as the church united, all believers could experience the glory of God!

As Doug continued ministering throughout our nation, I no longer had to make every trip. My nursing duties diminished. My most critical responsibility ended with the removal of the PICC line. Talk about freedom—not just for him, but for me, too. However, I still made all of those special meals and nutritional drinks for Doug. He let me know he intended to have a cheat day soon with all kinds of treats and planned to enjoy every bite of it.

Doug showed no signs of stopping or slowing down. He had renewed strength and was excited about the people he was partnering with for kingdom purposes. At the close of the Response Florida, Doug took the microphone and thanked everyone for joining the prayer gathering. He believed God had heard the cries of His people. God knew we would be there long before that day, in that place, in that appointed time.

As generational, denominational, and racial lines were crossed, Doug declared that what God had done would not stay there, but would reverberate across the city, state, nation, and the world. He asked that, without instruments, we express our adoration for that one name by singing "There's Something About that Name" by Bill and Gloria Gaither. If you are unfamiliar with the song, look it up. In the middle of your storm, sing it and believe it. In your good times, sing it and appreciate it. In the middle of your mourning, sing it and know that it is not over. There truly is something about that name! The song begins:

> Jesus, Jesus, Jesus; there's just something about that name.
> Master, Savior, Jesus, like the fragrance after the rain.

On November 10, we went back to MD Anderson for the results of the last set of tests. I had butterflies in my stomach and felt a bit anxious. I knew what we believed for, but the reality is that a number of thoughts ran through my mind. Doug confessed that his mind raced as well. This wasn't a matter of not believing that God had healed Doug. It was a matter of what the journey looked like from here on out.

Tears of gratitude streamed down my face as we learned that Doug was officially in remission. The latest PET scan showed no evidence of disease. Remission, whether partial or complete, means that the signs and symptoms of cancer are reduced. Some cancer cells can remain in the body for many years after treatment.

We would return to the hospital every three months for the first year to confirm that cancer was not in his body. After the first year of clean scans, Doug would go in for testing twice a year and, eventually, once a year until he completed five years of clean scans. We knew that the Great Physician had heard the prayers of our friends and spiritual family around the world and blessed all of us with the testimony of His healing power.

After we'd had all our questions answered, Doug thanked the doctor for his and the medical team's care and attention during his treatment then asked if he could pray for him. In that prayer, Doug stated that God had destined Dr. Westin to do what he does, to bring hope to the lives of desperate patients and their families. In all the times we'd shared our faith, the doctor had never responded like he did that day, bowing his head, closing his eyes, and even saying, "Amen," at the close of the prayer.

As we left the hospital, Doug constantly stopped, engaged people in conversation, and then asked if he could pray for them, never missing an opportunity to pray for patients and their families. Doug always does what he loves to do: telling people about Jesus and praying with and for people and their needs.

As we walked toward the parking garage, Doug told me that we must stay in a season of thanksgiving. "I don't just want to be healed," he said. "I want to be made whole in the Lord."

In Luke 17:11–19, Jesus healed ten lepers, but only one returned to thank Him.

Jesus asked, "Were not all ten cleansed? Where are the other nine? Has no one returned to give praise to God except this foreigner?" Then he said to him, "Rise and go; your faith has made you well."   (Luke 17:17–19 NIV)

Once home, I immediately gathered the communion elements so our family could partake together during this landmark moment in our family story. Ashley and Doug kneeled. She prayed over her father, spoke words of life over him, and declared God's goodness over his life. That tender scene will be forever ingrained in my memory. The season of mandatory hospital visits, infusions, and routine tests was over. We were so thankful, but didn't have much time to let it sink in until after an evening ministry gathering we'd committed to attend.

When we got home, Ashley went to her bedroom, Doug went to ours, and I went to our home office. Each of us needed our own private time in His presence. It was the perfect ending to a great day.

Doug has said, "The success of a leader is not just what you see on the platform, but in the unseen places where burdens are carried and dreams and visions are formed, causing restless and sometimes sleepless nights for the ones they are called to serve."

DETERMINED TO FINISH THE RACE WELL

I have seen Doug burn the midnight fuel in prayer and intercession for our nation and leaders, prayer requests he has been given, and more. I've seen him press in when I couldn't keep my eyes open if my life depended on it. He has more energy than the Energizer bunny, even in the season of battling cancer. I realize it is God's grace on his life, the desire to finish the race well, and the need to complete the task the Lord Jesus has put in front of him. That is what keeps him going.

Doug, like most men, is a bottom-line guy. He is slow and easy, while I am fast and steady. I see humor in the couples who are like us: opposites yet compatible. He is black and white, while I am full color. We laugh when I tell him up front that I need him to hear me in full color, occasionally throwing in special effects.

Sometimes, though, I discern that my conversation with him needs to be black and white. Doing that has enabled Doug to open up and share with me that he felt survivor's guilt. I paid close attention since I felt the same thing, except I was hurting for the spouses of those who'd been called to their eternal home.

We lost too many friends within a short amount of time. Pastor Dusty Kemp's home-going hit Doug hard. Not long ago, we had prayed together in a waiting area of MD Anderson, both of them there as patients. Dusty had preached a powerful sermon on a Sunday morning, had a great day with his wife, went to bed that evening, and woke up in the presence of the Lord. Pastor Buddy Hicks had an aneurysm while preaching. And there were others who we greatly esteemed. Each of their home-going celebrations was beautiful, but Doug needed his handkerchief to wipe away tears. Since our season with cancer, he has become more sentimental and more aware that we all live on borrowed time.

Doug read the Word, prayed, talked to God, and found peace, as did I. We had to choose to hear only one voice, our heavenly Father's, in the midst of all the noise. Survivor's guilt is real for many people and for many reasons. It was a real experience for the both of us, a time of questioning, reflecting, and, like everything else, trusting God, who alone knows our appointed time.

More than ever, we determined to rise every morning and say, "Thank You, Lord," no matter what the night had been like, no matter what trial or challenge would come. We resolved to never take life for granted, nor overlook an opportunity to be a life-giver to someone in need. A song Ashley wrote when she was twelve says, "Remember to always share a simple smile." Our desire now is to encourage others along the way and remind those facing battles that God is more than able.

I despise cancer and what it does to people. It is not prejudiced, it has no gender preference, and it doesn't respect age. It's an equal opportunity offender. Cancer may be the diagnosis, but it doesn't have to belong to us. I witnessed Doug pray for many in the last days of their battle with this dreaded disease.

While being interviewed for the documentary that Mike May was putting together, Pastor Rusty Griffin said, "Oftentimes, the word cancer brings in a spirit of fear and a spirit of death often comes with it. At times, the spirit of death takes us out before the cancer actually does."

Don't let fear set in and take you out. Discouragement from your diagnosis, test results, and distractions of all kinds have caused some to forget the Lord's visions and dreams for them. Doug says, "God is leading you through the process so that you may possess your promise. Don't lose hope!"

If you feel like giving up because your situation seems like too much to bear, spend a few hours sitting in a waiting room at a cancer hospital like MD Anderson. You will find people, young and old, who are fighting for their lives. Vanity goes out the window when you lose your hair, physical strength, and the ability to do simple things for yourself. Some patients have limbs missing, large tumors on their face, or parts of their skull missing. Yes, some are ready to quit. The battle has been intense and, in many cases, too long. But there are many who want to live and are doing everything in their power to overcome this dreaded disease.

HOLD ON TO GOD AND DON'T GIVE UP

As bad as your situation may seem, God is more than able to make a way. Sometimes life's challenges hardly seem worth fighting for, persevering through, or putting up with. We become overwhelmed and think it would be easier to be in our heavenly home. Don't give up. Press in and hold on to the One who will never leave you or forsake you. Keep your eyes on your destination and remember that God is not finished with you yet.

> AS BAD AS YOUR SITUATION MAY SEEM, GOD IS MORE THAN ABLE TO MAKE A WAY. DON'T GIVE UP. PRESS IN AND HOLD ON TO THE ONE WHO WILL NEVER LEAVE YOU OR FORSAKE YOU.

I've learned more than I could ever have imagined during our journey with cancer. It was a season of stretching, growing, faith-building, testing, and testimony sharing. It reminded me to never take for granted my health, finances, blessings, freedom, family, or friends.

I will remember to pray for healing for those who walk through the doors of MD Anderson and similar hospitals. I will pray for the caregivers to be strengthened as they endure their own emotional trials, being stretched physically and probably financially as well. But more than anything, I will pray for God to comfort those in need of their Father's embrace, for those who don't know the great I Am so they may encounter His love, peace, and healing touch.

Again, I say, "Thank you," to all who have prayed and continue to pray for us, sowing into our lives in every way possible and encouraging us along the way. Your love is a price-less treasure.

As life's unexpected detours come, may you maneuver through them with His grace and peace. And may your desire to win be greater than your moment of challenge.

EPILOGUE

It has been almost five years since the diagnosis and subsequent healing. Doug is scheduled to return soon to MD Anderson for blood work, a CT scan, and a follow-up appointment with Dr. Jason Westin. We believe we will hear that he is cancer-free; this year (2020) will complete the five-year waiting period in which each clean scan indicates that the patient is "in remission." Some doctors only use the word "cured" to describe people who've been in remission for a long time, often five years or more. In some people, lymphoma never completely goes away; this is where our trust in the Lord must shine through, no matter what the outcome.

All of these years later, with every scheduled appointment, it's still a battle of the mind. We continue to declare the Word of God over our lives and do our best not to allow our vain imagination to take over. There are days, and sometimes weeks, when

Doug seems to have to fight through the challenges of fatigue. In those times, he takes precautions to try to avoid any cold or flu bug that's going around.

While writing this book, I began to feel pain in my neck and some swelling in my lymph nodes—on the right side, just like Doug. I was in constant discomfort for a short season. I wondered if it was a spiritual attack, yet I felt that sharing our story could encourage others amid their storms. I was also hopeful that people who don't know God would be curious about Him and perhaps drawn to Him. Testimonies encourage others and that is what I wanted to do, knowing God would do the rest.

A thermography exam indicated I had swollen nodes in my neck and head. I was concerned, but kept writing our story and contending for my healing in prayer. In the meantime, I had more tests done and blood work showed no signs of cancer. It took some time for the discomfort to go away and the nodes to heal. I still feel the swelling on occasion and it makes me reflect on our trials and triumphs.

In his end-of-the-year message for 2014, Doug wrote, "It's a good time and opportunity for hitting our reset buttons. A time for recalibration, realignments, resolving, reviving, rebuilding, restoring, refreshing, reshuffling, and getting a renewed revelation of God's purposes for our lives and relationships."

That message is an excellent reminder to all of us on any given day. I am grateful that we realigned and recalibrated, so that months later, when we received Doug's diagnosis, we could be strong in the Lord to allow the restoring, rebuilding, and reviving of healthy cells in his body to take place.

Interestingly, that message, in retrospect, was a word not just for others, but for us and what we were getting ready to encounter. Recently, Doug was talking about our 2015 joys and challenges at a gathering of pastors and leaders. To borrow from Charles Dickens' *A Tale of Two Cities*, "It was the best of times, it was the worst of times..." While it was one of our most physically and mentally challenging years, it was also one of the most practically and spiritually impacting years in the ministry. There is still great fruit being born and lives impacted from that season.

Everyone goes through life-altering experiences, whether tragedy, sudden loss, or temporary setbacks. In time, with the support and prayers of those around us, we regain hope and trust where it had been lost or hidden. Doug has always encouraged us that even though challenges, obstacles, and life-altering events occur, God is there for us with His arms outstretched. His unfailing love will see us through and His plan for our lives hasn't changed.

> NO MATTER WHAT YOU'RE GOING THROUGH, GOD HAS NOT FORGOTTEN YOU. HE HAS A PLAN AND A PURPOSE FOR YOU. HIS WORD OVER YOUR LIFE IS TRUE AND HE WILL BE FAITHFUL TO COMPLETE IT.

No matter what you're going through, Doug and I want you to remember that God has not forgotten you. He has a plan and a purpose for you that is far greater than any of the temporary circumstances that may be plaguing you. His Word over your life is true and He will be faithful to complete it. Rest, as we have, in His love.

Every single moment you are thinking of me! How precious and wonderful to consider that you cherish me constantly in your every thought! O God, your desires toward me are more than the grains of sand on every shore! When I awake each morning, you're still with me.

(Psalm 139:17–18 TPT)

ABOUT THE AUTHOR

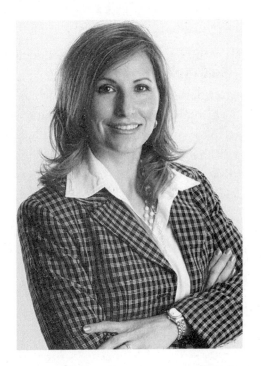

Lisa Stringer is the wife of Doug Stringer, the founder and president of Somebody Cares America/International, a network of organizations impacting their communities through unified grassroots efforts.

Lisa worked in the secular radio and music entertainment industry for seventeen years, becoming the first female program director of a top-40 station in a major market in the United States. Later, she became the vice president of programming and promotions of a radio group. Lisa has received numerous awards, including gold and platinum records for her contribution to the success of many highly recognizable recording artists and entertainers.

She homeschooled her daughter, Ashley, who is now enrolled in dual programs at a local community college and working on the release of her second EP.

Lisa travels with Doug as they minister to many around the globe, ranging from those of the persecuted church to those suffering in the aftermath of human tragedy, such as the Haitian earthquake, the tsunami in Japan, and Hurricane Dorian in the Bahamas. Lisa enjoys opportunities where she has been able to interpret for her husband as they minister throughout Central and South America. She and her husband are also regular guests on various television programs that air throughout the world.

Lisa has a heart for the less fortunate, widows, and orphans. She has served on various boards and has traveled to over thirty-four nations.

The Stringers live in the greater Houston area.

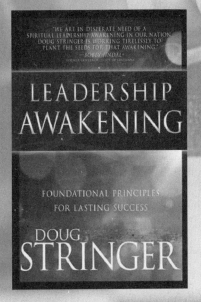

TOGETHER RESCUING LIVES

**PRAYER INITIATIVES • COMPASSION EVANGELISM
DISASTER RESPONSE•LEADERSHIP DEVELOPMENT**

Join us in reaching
the hurting, restoring hope,
and reviving hearts—
showing others we care
because Jesus cares!

**For more information or to donate,
visit SomebodyCares.org
or follow us on
Facebook and Twitter
@_SomebodyCares**

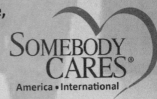

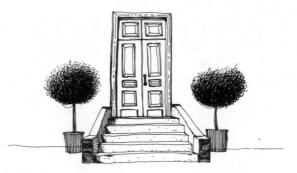

Welcome to Our House!

We Have a Special Gift for You

It is our privilege and pleasure to share in your love of Christian books. We are committed to bringing you authors and books that feed, challenge, and enrich your faith.

To show our appreciation, we invite you to sign up to receive a specially selected **Reader Appreciation Gift**, with our compliments. Just go to the Web address at the bottom of this page.

God bless you as you seek a deeper walk with Him!

WE HAVE A GIFT FOR YOU. VISIT:

whpub.me/nonfictionthx

WHITAKER
HOUSE